Health
Motivations

ALSO BY CAROL M. MORGAN
AND DORAN J. LEVY, PH.D.

Segmenting the Mature Market
and
*Marketing to the Mindset of Boomers
and Their Elders*

Health Motivations

7 Dimensions That Shape America's Health

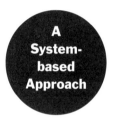

A
System-
based
Approach

Carol M. Morgan *and* Doran J. Levy, Ph.D.

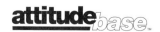

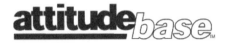

66 Ninth Street East, Suite 1407
Saint Paul, MN 55101
651-228-7250

Cover design by 45 Degrees/Minneapolis

Library of Congress Catalog Number: 2011961328

ISBN: 978-0-9705605-0-6

1. Health 2. Motivations 3. Segmentations 4. Attitude measurement

Health Motivations is available at special discounts for bulk purchases by corporations, institutions, and other organizations. For more information, please contact us at 651-228-7250 or email: cmorgan@strategicdirectionsgroup.com.

ACKNOWLEDGEMENTS

Shaping this book was facilitated by the insights offered by Donald R. Wright, Ph.D., Doris E. Wright, Julie S. Fine, M.P.H., M.S.W., and James Delmont, Ph.D. We thank them for their suggestions, many of which we incorporated. Their comments proved invaluable in organizing the book's content, as well as increasing its usefulness.

We also wish to thank Edward M. Morgan for his work managing the extensive data collection and analysis efforts on our studies of the U.S. mature market.

John G. Morgan, M.S. was the principal architect of the Morgan-Levy Health Cube computer system. His contribution to its creation was extremely valuable.

Although our original study in 1989 was self-funded, we appreciate the participation of 30 major corporations in the syndicated studies that followed. These corporations enabled us to gather the millions of pieces of data we analyzed in order to create the Morgan-Levy Health Cube system, as well as this book.

Finally, we wish to express our gratitude to the late William Stephenson, Ph.D., whose life-work had a profound influence on our efforts to better understand human motivation.

TABLE
of CONTENTS

PART 3

PART 4

APPENDICES

INDICES

LIST
of FIGURES

PART I

Chapter 1

A NEW PERSPECTIVE

An avalanche of costs

Everyone knows the problem. The cost of health care in the U.S. threatens to overwhelm our economy. Over the past few decades, various solutions have been proposed and implemented to deal with these skyrocketing costs. And yet costs continue to escalate. They do so in great part because consumers make choices on a daily basis that have or will have detrimental effects on their health.

Motivations deliver results

This book's fundamental premise is that by knowing an individual's health-related motivations in detail, targeted health-messages can be developed and delivered. These messages, in turn, will increase the possibility that an individual will make more healthful choices in the future.

A radically different approach

While we can tally the results of the destructive health-care decisions we make every day, and can isolate the behaviors themselves, what remains difficult to pinpoint is *why* we choose to make unhealthful choices. What are the motivations behind these choices?

Unique multi-dimensional view

After establishing seven key attitudinal dimensions, this book goes on to show how these attitudes relate to demographics and behaviors. In bringing attitudes, demographics, and behaviors together, we provide a unique and multi-faceted perspective on what drives health-care choices.

Our book is not a view in time of the health of the mature market. Instead, it is structured to show relationships between our attitudinal dimensions and more conventional measurements.

Our interest is not in reporting the number of persons 40 and older who have a particular disease. Instead, we isolate the behaviors and demographics of someone who, for example, believes he or she is Able to Understand Health Information, one of our key attitudinal dimensions. Does a person who suffers from a chronic disease score lower on Trust in Doctors, another dimension?

Achieving three goals

As experts in motivational research, we believe that by isolating and understanding these motivations three important goals can be achieved. The comprehensive understanding of health attitudes delivered by the Morgan-Levy Health Cube would prove highly useful in budgeting and planning communication programs. A decision could be made to identify and target those more receptive to modifying their health-related attitudes and, by extension, their behaviors.

Secondly, usable insights into individual motivations would also result in programs and products being

3

produced reflecting those motivations. And, finally, it will be possible to produce health communications targeted to an individual, complementing that person's motivations, that is, his or her mind set.

These communications, far more targeted than any produced today, would engage more persons or patients to actualize their own positive health-related motivations. And today's technology can facilitate the production and dissemination of such targeted health-communications.

Engagement drives change

Why make this effort? Research has shown that the more a piece of communication reflects a person's motivations and interests, the more it will engage that person. The precise alignment of communication messages to individual motivations will yield improved results.

Whether doctors or pharmaceutical marketers, pharmacists or wellness counselors, those involved in the delivery of health-care services and products will recognize the benefit of being able to cost-effectively, accurately, and quickly measure the motivations driving health-related behaviors.

We developed the Morgan-Levy Health Cube precisely to offer significant benefits that can be applied to strategic planning, program development, and communication strategies.

An Internet-based system

The Morgan-Levy Health Cube is completed over the Internet; its questions are self-administered. The cost of using it are far lower than employing a highly paid professional who most likely will spend hours asking probing questions to achieve the same type of results. The Morgan-Levy Health Cube uses a stan-

4

dardized process. On an individual level, it generates reports on each dimension comparing the participant to the general U.S. population 40 and older. In aggregate, various populations and subpopulations can be compared. Comparisons can also be made between responses given at different times.

A comprehensive viewpoint

It is true health-related motivations have been previously explored. However, these studies and programs have typically focused on one dimension.

We believe human motivations are complex and cannot be explained from one perspective. At times, these one dimensional probes into health-related motivations have also been developed from very small samples.

In contrast, the motivations captured in our seven independent health-related dimensions present a far more comprehensive perspective on the impediments to better health.

Decades of research

Having collected data on 20,000 persons 40 and older over the past two decades using extensive questionnaires, we have spent the past five years on its analysis. We brought 50 years of experience in creating attitudinally based segmentation studies for major U.S. corporations to our study of the 40 and older U.S. population and its health-related motivations.

Two approaches

The result of our efforts is the Morgan-Levy Health Cube, which incorporates our seven critical motivational dimensions and facilitates their mass application and use.

5

While our Internet-based system facilitates the formal and scientific use of the Morgan-Levy Health Cube, the insights this book presents can also be used in an informal and intuitive way.

Complementing the seven key dimensions are our three health-related segmentations which give additional perspectives and depth to our dimensions.

Dimensions critical to good health

After describing America's surging health-care costs, our book delineates the seven health-care motivational dimensions forming the basis of the Morgan-Levy Health Cube. It also provides information supporting the importance of each dimension to our good health. Our three health-related segmentations are then explored. These chapters are followed by a description showing the extent to which the seven critical health-care dimensions are found in each of our segments.

The book goes on to show how our insights benefit not only the individual, but can also be applied to various types of health communications, marketing efforts, and strategic decisions, to everything from one-on-one interviews to large databases to program design. An appendix contains sections supporting our system's validity and reliability.

Chapter 2

THE HEALTH-CARE AVALANCHE

Costs threaten our economy

Like an avalanche thundering down a mountainside burying everything in its path, America's health-care costs are threatening to overwhelm our economy. Experts differ on the weight they assign to each possible cause of this avalanche and what can be done to divert its massive impact. Virtually everyone agrees, however, that health-care costs are out of control.

Paul Ginsburg, president of the Center for Studying Health System Change (HSC) believes soaring health-care costs "just can't go on much longer."[1] "The health insurance system in the United States is broken . . . ," says Regina E. Herzlinger, professor of business administration at the Harvard Business School. "The situation," she believes, "is dire."[2]

Increases in health-care spending

Our present predicament has been years in the making. In 1970 national health spending totaled

7

$74.3 billion. By 1980 health-care costs had more than tripled to $251.1 billion.[3] The next decade witnessed an almost tripling of health-care costs when $696 billion was spent in 1990.[4] Over the twenty years that followed, health-care spending tripled once again. The U.S. Department of Health and Human Services estimates that during 2010 total national spending on health care grew 3.9 percent and reached $2.5 trillion.[5]

As percent of GDP

Just over forty years ago in 1970 national health-care spending represented 7.4 percent of the gross domestic product (GDP), the total output of goods and services. By 1980 it had risen to 9.3 percent.[6] In 2000, national health-care spending reached 13.3 percent of GDP.[7] Forecasts from the Centers for Medicaid and Medicare Services (CMS), Office of the Actuary predict that that share will continue to rise, reaching 19.8 percent of GDP in 2020.[8] If this scenario proves true, in less than ten years health care will represent one dollar of every five of the total value of goods and services produced in the U.S.

In a speech given in 2003 Uwe E. Reinhardt, the noted health-care economist, predicted that by 2030, U.S. health-care expenditures would jump to 28 percent of GDP and to 40 percent in 2050. These estimates do not include the impact of aging baby boomers and their increased need for health-care. If boomers are included in these computations, he predicts health care could reach 46 percent of GDP by 2050.[9] Reinhardt's projections are echoed by the Congressional Budget Office (CBO) which estimates that health-care costs will reach 25 percent of GDP in 2025 and 37 percent in 2050.[10] Without significant changes to our health-care system, health care could become the dominant U.S. industry within the next few decades.

Pointing fingers

Many forces contribute to our immense health-cost spiral. Some experts underscore the escalating consumption of more expensive prescription drugs. New technological innovations are also blamed for pushing up the cost of health care. The threat of medical malpractice lawsuits and the actual costs of litigating them also adds to our health-care costs.

Other industry analysts stress that health care is a one-on-one service industry of "handcrafted" solutions which do not lend themselves to gains in productivity. Some suggest that increasing salaries for health-care workers have contributed to spiraling health-care costs, as has a rise in hospital spending.

With health-care services paid for by scores of health insurance companies, we continue to face an expensive administrative nightmare. Although more data is being collected electronically and shared with various entities, administrative costs remain immense.

And, finally, many fingers point to the consumer who wants the very best and latest treatments, with little idea of their cost. Consumers may demand procedures that offer little benefit relative to their cost, as well as rely on heroic, end-of-life measures which do not appreciably extend life. The consumer expects someone else to cover these expenses.

Consumers are responsible

"The people to blame in the end, the ones ultimately responsible, are consumers," says economist Christopher Thornberg, formerly of UCLA's *Anderson Forecast.* "People don't adequately take into account the true costs of the services they're consuming."[11]

Added to these causes for the increasing expenditures on health-care services is the reality of an aging population. Baby boomers, the oldest of whom are just

9

becoming eligible for Medicare, will push health-care expenditures to astronomical heights.

So far, solutions haven't worked

Trying to hang the blame for increasing health-care costs on one group or another or one cause or another continues because, according to Julie Appleby writing in *USA Today,* "no one really has an answer on how to slow the increases . . . . Everything tried in the past decade from wage and price controls under President Nixon to managed care has ultimately failed to stem rising costs."[12]

In his speech to the American RE Healthcare Symposium, Reinhardt confirmed that ". . . neither government nor businesses have found a way to tame health-care costs."[13] According to some experts, the hope of finding a solution seems slim. Appleby quotes Reinhardt himself as believing that "We should get used to the idea of double-digit health insurance increases for the next 10 to 20 years. I see no relief coming."[14]

Need to focus on consumer

If consumers are "ultimately responsible" for the increases in health-care services, as economist Thornberg believes, why not focus solutions on consumers? But the solutions proposed by economists and business gurus—from creating electronic patient records to standardizing the number of health plan types offered, from negotiating the price paid for pharmaceuticals to reducing duplication of care—typically do not focus on the patient.

Of the ten suggestions made by expert Karen Davis, president of The Commonwealth Fund, for controlling health-care costs, one takes up the consumer. Costs can be controlled, she believes, if "shared decision making by informed patients" is encouraged.[15] Of the six sug-

10

gestions made by Regina E. Herzlinger in order to put consumers, actually employees, "in charge of health-care," two focus on consumers: this group should be given "incentives to shop intelligently" and provided with "relevant information." The remaining suggestions have to do with product design and pricing.[16]

New emphasis needed

If we acknowledge that previous solutions to reducing health-care cost increases have not worked, we must look for solutions from a new perspective. But while placing much of the responsibility for increases in health-care costs on the consumer, both past and current solutions proposed by economists and business professors have not typically included changing consumer behavior in order to reduce expenditures.

Reducing health-care costs through prevention

Major corporations and health maintenance organizations (HMOs), however, are now increasing efforts to reduce health-care costs by encouraging employees to adopt healthier lifestyles. Studies have repeatedly shown that participation in various measures, from smoking cessation to weight reduction, exercise to compliance with treatment regimes, prevents health-care problems from developing or worsening. The National Business Group on Health reports that such "fitness programs for workers" are starting to "pay some dividends."[17]

Appealing to motivations

We maintain that all efforts at prevention would enjoy greater success if programs and communication were designed to appeal to specific segments defined

11

by their motivations and attitudes toward critical dimensions contributing to health. Understanding such motivations is especially critical in the mature population because U.S. consumers 40 and older are responsible for 72 percent of all health-care spending.[18]

Any positive change in the mature population's attitudes toward prevention and more healthful behaviors could result in great savings, as well as longer, healthier lives. For example, a study published in the *American Journal of Public Health* showed that if the prevalence of diabetes and high blood pressure were reduced by five percent, the U.S. would save $33.7 billion annually over the near and medium terms.[19]

REFERENCES

[1] David R. Francis. "Health care costs are up. Here are the culprits." *csmonitor.com*. Christian Science Monitor, 15 Dec. 2003. Web. 7 Oct. 2010.

[2] Regina E. Herzlinger. "Are Consumers the Cure for Broken Health Insurance?" *hbswk.hbs.edu*. Harvard Business School, Working Knowledge for Business Leaders, 5 Aug. 2002. Web. 12 Oct. 2010.

[3] Katharine R Levit, et al. "National Health Spending Trends, 1960-1993." *healthaffairs.org*. Health Affairs 13.5 (1994): 14-15. Web. 12 Oct. 2010.

[4] Levit, et al.

[5] Sean P. Keehan, et al. "National Health Spending Projections Through 2020: Economic Recovery and Reform Drive Faster Spending Growth." *healthaffairs.org*. Health Affairs 30.8 (2011):1594-1605. Web. 17 Oct. 2011.

[6] Levit, et al.

[7] Katharine R. Levit, et al. "Trends in U.S. Health Care Spending, 2001." *healthaffairs.org*. Health Affairs 22.1 (2003): 154-155. Web. 23 Nov. 2010.

[8] Keehan, et al.

[9] Uwe E. Reinhardt. Sum. American RE Healthcare Symposium 2003. *greenleaf-co.com*. Hyatt Regency Scottsdale Resort and Spa at Gainey Ranch, Scottsdale, AZ, 31 Mar. 2003. Keynote address. Web. 10 July 2010.

[10] "The Long-Term Outlook for Health Care Spending, Nov. 2007." The Congress of the United States, Congressional Budget Office. *cbo.gov*. Web. 10 July 2010.

[11] Julie Appleby. "Finger pointers can't settle on who's to blame for health costs." *usatoday.com*. USA Today, 20 Aug. 2002. Web. 10 July 2010.

[12] Appleby.

[13] Reinhardt.

[14] Appleby.

[15] Karen Davis. "Toward a High Performance Health System: the Commonwealth Fund's New Commission." *healthaffairs.org*. Health Affairs 24.5 (2005): 1356-60. Web. 10 July 2010.

[16] Regina E. Herzlinger. "Let's Put Consumers in Charge of Health Care." *hbr.org*. Harvard Business Review, July 2002, reprint RO207B: 1. Web. 15 Oct. 2010.

[17] "Corporate fitness programs create healthier employees." *allbusiness.com.* National Business Group on Health, 1 Jan. 2005. Web. 7 Oct. 2010.

[18] "Table 1, Total Health Services— Median and Mean Expenses per Person with Expense and Distribution of Expenses by Source of Payment: United States 2006." Medical Expenditure Panel Survey, Agency for Healthcare Research and Quality. *meps.ahrq.gov.* Web. 10 July 2010.

[19] "Disease Prevention Could Save U.S. Billions of Dollars Annually." Bloomberg Businessweek, 22 Nov. 2010. Web. 2 Nov. 2011.

Chapter 3

UNDERSTANDING MOTIVATIONS

Chronic disease crisis

While treating acute diseases now requires fewer of our health-care dollars, paying for chronic diseases, whether diabetes, emphysema, or heart disease, threatens to overwhelm the U.S. economy. The vast increase in the number of persons with one or more chronic diseases has prompted various entities, from employers to pharmaceutical companies, insurers to health professionals, to focus on the health choices made by consumers, employees, and patients.

All of these parties wish to motivate change that leads to better health. An employer hopes to see an employee losing weight, while a pharmaceutical company would like patients to adhere to a drug regimen treating glaucoma. Studies have repeatedly shown that "motivation is a very important intervening variable when evaluating health promotion and resulting behavior change."[1]

Values shape choices

Health-care choices are made based on underlying values. In one instance, a woman continues to smoke cigarettes because she wishes to remain slim. Being seen as a svelte fashionista is of greater importance to her than having healthy lungs. A man makes a habit of drinking several alcoholic drinks each evening with friends because he places a greater importance on the social aspect of drinking than on the damage alcohol is doing to his body.

Another woman can't find the time for a checkup because she is too busy caring for her family. She values providing care to her family more than taking care of herself. A motorcyclist never wears a helmet when he rides. He values freedom, the sensation of wind whipping through his hair, far more than safeguarding his health.

In contrast, a 72-year-old man who has already had one heart attack believes he can preserve and improve his health by walking vigorously for three miles a day without fail. He is motivated to be as healthy as possible, even as he ages. A woman eats a low-fat diet because she wishes to do whatever she can to avoid the cardiovascular disease that struck down her mother.

Each of these persons has made a health-related choice based on his or her values. The motivation to do something or avoid it springs from these values. Personal values impel motivation.

Attitudes reveal values

Such values are internal; they reside within us. We can grasp an individual's values only when they are revealed through some external expression: an attitude. These expressions can include a behavior or a verbal or written statement.

As scholars have noted, "attitudes have an impact

16

on health experience. They may affect health either positively or negatively. In order to affect attitude change towards a given health issue existing attitudes have to be determined." [2]

While some believe we can decipher a person's values through their behaviors, we believe doing so can be misleading. Intuitive leaps from behaviors to values are highly unreliable.

For example, if we see a woman applying sunscreen everyday we could conclude she values health. We observe the behavior and ascribe her unwavering application to an underlying value of lowering her risk of developing melanoma. However, in this case if we asked the woman why she uses sunscreen she will tell us that she does so because she is committed to looking as young as possible. Using sunscreen helps her avoid liver spots, as well as wrinkling and sagging. What we intuit as her underlying value may not be in any way that which impels her behavior.

We believe people can articulate the values that motivate them to behave in a certain way. This expression may be aided by the skills of a trained interviewer using various techniques, such as laddering. Specific methodologies have also been developed that avoid some of the problems of using scales, such as lying or distorting the truth.

In the case of our fashion-conscious woman, she may agree with the attitude statement "If I had to choose between being slim and being healthy, I'd choose slim." Her agreement with this attitude reveals her underlying value: she values slimness over health. Her agreement with this statement is a tangible external representation of a value she holds. With this insight, we know the all-important *why* behind her behavior. We can now develop targeted messages and strategies based on it.

Change a possibility

Will our fashionista ever exhibit a different behavior? Will she ever give up cigarettes? It may be that she values giving birth to a healthy baby more than she values being slim. In this case, when she becomes pregnant, one value supersedes another. She quits smoking in order to protect her unborn child, something she sees as a greater good. Recognizing that our fashion maven can be motivated to quit smoking if the health of her unborn child is stressed, her doctor can provide messages supporting this value. She could be directed to a smoking cessation program designed specifically for pregnant women, one that recognizes and ties into maternal concern for the baby's health.

Individual values needed

While our fashionista exhibits a value, an underlying concern for her child, we cannot assume that all pregnant women who smoke share the same value. While establishing and understanding attitudes and the motivations that spring from them, it is also necessary to recognize that effective motivation messages and programs must be targeted to the individual. Any program based on the idea that members of a class or group, whether pregnant women or diabetics, share the same motivations will be less than successful.

Targeted messages effective

In order to provide the communication and support that will inspire the hoped-for change, what motivates each individual must be understood. By understanding individual motivations, targeted appeals can be made and tailored programs constructed. Advertisers and marketers concluded long ago that the closer a message is to an individual's own values, the more effective the communication.

18

Virtually everyone has had the experience of being given health-related information so inappropriate to one's values that the communication is jarring. For example, a proactive patient committed to a healthful lifestyle finds herself being lectured to by a doctor who lays out threatening scenarios if the patient "doesn't do something." The doctor fails to connect with the motivations of a patient already committed to "doing something." The patient is put off by a message that doesn't relate to her values. Such mismatched messages can result in hostility toward the doctor, a lack of compliance, and poorer health.

Care and motivations

Motivations are not only important in preventing disease and managing it optimally when it occurs, but also in the provision of care. The current emphasis on holistic healthcare and on patient-centered care underscores the importance of a patient's or health-care consumer's values and beliefs.

In patient-centered care, for example, these values and beliefs are to be defined, understood, and incorporated into the relationship between provider and patient, as well as the treatment plan. Health-care choices, made on the basis of those values, impact not only the patient's health, but also the nation's health-care expenditures.

Assessing motivations

Since understanding the patient's "values" are at the very center of such an approach, how are such values to be assessed and established? Recent studies illustrating the benefits of motivational interviews have appeared in scholarly journals. One study, for example, on the use of such interviews in an ophthalmology clinic showed that they were cost-effective and improved compliance.[3]

19

Interviews too costly

Today there are 138 million persons 40 and older in the U.S. By 2030 that number will increase to 180 million. Conducting motivational interviews, regardless of their intrinsic value, becomes astronomically expensive.

The cost of conducting motivational interviews is driven in part by the need for highly trained interviewers. It is important to note that the usefulness and reliability of motivational interviews rests on the training and experience of those conducting them. And the more highly trained the interviewer, usually the more highly paid.

In contrast, the Internet-based Morgan-Levy Health Cube system is a quick, reliable, and cost-effective way of assessing and defining the health-related motivations of those 40 and older. Self-administered, its use requires no trained professional. The brief process can be completed at home, in a doctor's office, or at work.

Results inevitably filtered

In addition, even a well-trained interviewer committed to remaining objective will still see an employee or patient through his or her own eyes. It is possible the way the interview is conducted or the interviewer's conclusions about a person may be colored in some way.

For example, a researcher using the Implicit Associations Test (IAT) surveyed 400 health professionals attending the annual meeting of the North American Association for the Study of Obesity (NAASO). The researcher found that those surveyed "considered fat people lazier, more stupid, and more worthless than their thinner counterparts."[4] Other studies of primary care physicians and nurses have revealed similar views.

Unbiased and reliable

The Morgan-Levy Health Cube offers a standard-ized process for determining health-related motiva-tions. Unlike the potential prejudicial filters of individ-ual interviewers, the Morgan-Levy Health Cube system asks the same questions of each participant. Each question has been carefully written to avoid bias of any type. These questions were developed through exten-sive research described in the following chapter.

In Appendix A we present data supporting the reli-ability of our system. In its effectiveness and effi-ciency, we believe the Morgan-Levy Health Cube meets criteria established by the International Organi-zation for Standardization (ISO) for a usable product.

A time-consuming approach

But besides the immense cost of conducting moti-vation interviews on the 40 and older population and the need for trained interviewers, there are other prob-lems as well. Motivational interviews take time, whether one session is needed or several. Today health-care professionals are under considerable time pres-sure. The typical doctor visit lasts an average of just 22 minutes.[5]

During these very few minutes a doctor, who must now be trained in motivational interviewing skills, will have to not only listen attentively to his patient's com-plaints and symptoms, develop a diagnosis, and suggest a course of treatment, but also analyze his or her pa-tient's motivations. In addition, the patient or employee may lack the time for a motivational interview.

Impossible to generalize

Regardless of the interviewer's skill, conclusions from a motivational interview cannot be generalized

21

from an individual interview to entire databases. Motivational interviews do not allow us to collect standardized data and draw conclusions from them regarding defined populations.

The Morgan-Levy Health Cube system, in contrast, gives those involved in health-care products and services the ability to compare an individual to those within any group. Everyone who has ever been or will ever be classified by our system is asked the same questions in the same way. Because of this, data sets can be compared.

Measuring, quantifying change

Our system can also deliver another key benefit. It can quickly and easily measure changes in a person's health-related attitudes.

Persons who have been classified using our system can be retested at some later time. Doing so will show if there has been movement up or down one or more of the seven critical health-care dimensions measured by the Morgan-Levy Health Cube system.

If health-related attitudes have changed, we can then examine behaviors. Have these attitudinal changes resulted in motivating people to adopt new behaviors? An example of our system's ability to measure motivational change over time is seen in Appendix B which addresses the validity of our system. That chapter shows changes in attitudes linked to statistically significant changes in behavior.

REFERENCES

[1] R.B. Kelly, et al. "Prediction of motivation and behavior change following health promotion: role of health beliefs, social support, and self-efficacy." *ncbi.nlm.nih.gov.* Social Science and Medicine 32.3 (1991): 311-2. Web. 28 Jan. 2011.

[2] R.M. Cross. "Exploring attitudes: the case for Q methodology." *her.oxfordjournals.org.* Health Education Research 20.2 (2004): 206-213. Web. 16 July 2011.

[3] P.F. Cook, et al. "Feasibility of motivational interviewing delivered by a glaucoma educator to improve medication adherence." *ncbi.nlm.nih.gov.* Clinical Ophthalmology 4 (2010): 1091-101. Web. 25 Dec. 2010.

[4] Jason Zengerle. "Big Trouble." *The New Republic* 19 Nov. 2007: 24-27. Print.

[5] Lena M. Chen, et al. "Primary Care Visit Duration and Quality." *archinte.ama-assn.rg.* Archives of Internal Medicine 169.20 (2009): 1866-72. Web. 7 July 2010.

Chapter 4

CREATING OUR HEALTH CUBE SYSTEM

The system, its benefits

In the previous chapter, we stressed the importance of understanding health-related attitudes in shaping optimal messages and programs to motivate change. We also showed that the process of deciphering consumer attitudes about health can be expensive, lengthy, and complicated. We created the Morgan-Levy Health Cube system to capture the attitudes behind consumers' health choices quickly, inexpensively, and simply by translating our research into an Internet-based system.

The Morgan-Levy Health Cube is based on extensive studies we conducted on the U.S. population 40 and older over a period of 20 years. The large random samples of the U.S. population we used to derive our system were consistent with the U.S. population based on income, age, gender and region of the country.

These studies provided the data from which we created the three separate psychographic or attitudinal segmentations described in Part Three of this book. Each attitudinal segmentation focuses on a separate aspect of health by the 40 and older population: general perspectives, views related to the acquisition of health information, and, finally, positions on compliance with treatment and wellness plans. Because our system presents a multi-dimensional view based on these three different aspects of health, we decided to refer to it as a cube.

The seven critical dimensions we describe in this book are derived from the perspective of these three segmentations. These seven dimensions can be used on their own or in conjunction with segments within our three separate segmentations. Each segment is motivated to a greater or lesser degree on each of the seven dimensions.

An examination of segments within one of our segmentations, whether Health, Health Information, or Health Compliance, reveals how persons 40 and older in the U.S. population group themselves by the level of importance they place on the issues measured by the dimensions.

For example, later in the book we will see that Proactives, one of our Health segments, score high on the Healthy Lifestyle dimension. In contrast, Uninvolved Fatalists, one of our Health Information segments, score exceptionally low on this dimension.

These segmentations and a raft of behaviors and demographics were explored in our two previous books: *Segmenting the Mature Market* and *Marketing to the Mindset of Boomers and Their Elders.*

Proprietary measurement system

Since 1988 our work, including the research that forms the basis of the Morgan-Levy Health Cube, has been based on a proprietary attitude measurement system. We believe the process used in the traditional approach to attitude measurement often fails to engage

25

the respondent. The boredom of answering scores of attitude statements can lead the respondent to misrepresent his or her motivations. In addition, the traditional approach to attitude measurement allows respondents to answer positively or negatively to all the statements.

The scores of attitude statements we used in creating our three psychographic segmentations reflected insights from focus groups we conducted, as well as perspectives gathered from secondary research. From these we extracted the key issues the attitude statements address. Because redundancy is crucial to fully understanding motivations, we focused on the critical issues from several different angles. We also limited the attitude statements to those on which action could be taken, if not by the respondent, then by another person or organization. These attitude statements were used in lengthy questionnaires on large samples of persons 40 and older.

Making choices, revealing attitudes

Unlike the traditional approach, the methodology we use is structured so that respondents reveal their innermost feelings about the issues under investigation. Typically respondents are presented with key attitude statements on cards and then asked to rank order the statements as to those with which they agree strongly, agree somewhat, disagree strongly, disagree somewhat, or feel neutral about. They then place their rankings on a grid restricting their selection in each of the five categories.

This process forces respondents to prioritize what is important to them. Because the statements are ranked and their position on the grid is restricted, it is far more difficult for respondents to misrepresent their true feelings. In our view, the approach we use better reflects the real world, a world in which choices must be made:

we cannot have everything.

The methodology we use compares one person against every other person. If, for example, one individual wants to hide an attitude in the neutral pile and others vehemently disagree with the statement, we have an insight into the person giving the neutral score. Since the respondent doesn't know how others will rate the statement, he or she indirectly reveals hidden feelings.

Participants may feel positive, negative, or neutral about statements such as "Exercising four times a week takes too much time" or "Reducing the amount of salt I use in my food is not a difficult thing to do." By comparing the respondents' rankings on scores of statements, we are able to differentiate groups, or segments, which feel differently on various key dimensions of the issues under investigation. The creation of each dimension that is part of the Morgan-Levy Health Cube began with this sorting process.

A 360° perspective

From the data we collected, we extracted the attitudes forming both our three separate health-related segmentations, as well as the seven key dimensions found in the Morgan-Levy Health Cube. The sophisticated mathematical methodology we use assesses the attitudinal data, revealing the segments and dimensions at the center of our work. These psychographic aspects can then be compared to respondents' behaviors and demographics, as well as to their Internet and media usage. In this way, we learn not only what people do, but *why* they do it.

In this book, we will show how our system can be used in a variety of ways, from evaluating patients in a doctor's office to determining employee attitudes, from designing public health programs to use in market re-

27

search for health-related products and services.

Our history

In the 1960s and 1970s Doran Levy, one of the firm's principals, studied under William Stephenson, a renowned physicist and psychologist. Stephenson had studied at University College London under Charles Spearman, a pioneer of factor analysis. Stephenson is best known for his invention of Q-methodology. The purpose of Q-methodology is "to reveal subjective structures, attitudes, and perspectives from the standpoint of the person or persons being observed."[1]

In 1976, Levy co-founded what was to become Strategic Directions Group, a firm specializing in attitudinal or psychographic segmentation for marketing research purposes. Building on Stephenson's methods, Levy developed a series of analytic techniques to understand the motivations behind individuals' choices.

Diverse experience

Strategic Directions Group conducts proprietary studies for large companies using the methodology we've described. Our work spans multiple industries, including pharmaceutical, medical devices, food products, travel, credit cards, investments, insurance, banking, home products, home building and gasoline purchases.

Because segmentation studies require significant samples and high-level analysis, they are major projects most often funded by large organizations. Once clients understand the motivations of their customers, as well as their demographics and buying behaviors, they are able to formulate optimal marketing strategies, craft products people want, and target advertising messages.

The application of these techniques to health-care

issues was of particular interest to Carol M. Morgan. As the director of public relations at Hennepin County Medical Center, a major teaching hospital in Minnesota, Morgan experienced the U.S. health system in action. Later, after forming her own marketing firm, Morgan worked with a wide range of companies involved in various facets of health care.

Long-term studies on health

We began our studies on those 40 and older in the U.S. market because we believed an attitudinal or psychographic segmentation perspective could add a great deal to the understanding of mature consumers. At that time, most markets, including this one, were viewed in terms of demographics. To a large extent, this demographic perspective prevails even today.

Many mass marketers assume the attitudes of all of those in their 50s are the same; that all 70-year-olds are driven by identical motivations. While demographic data presents only a partial perspective, it is easy to collect and analyze, as well as to understand and apply.

In contrast, the figure on the next page illustrates how defining a group of people by their attitudes and then linking the resulting segments to demographics and behaviors, such as Internet and media usage, provides a 360° perspective, an accurate and actionable blueprint. It is true that attitudinal data is typically proprietary and more expensive to develop. The Morgan-Levy Health Cube itself is based on a massive investment not only on data collection and processing, but also on years of analysis.

While many articles and books now address the impact of our aging population on the cost of health care and our economy in general, the inexorable and undeniable aging of our population has been noted for half a century. For example, in 1958, Robert D. Dodge pre-

ORGANIZING AROUND MOTIVATIONS

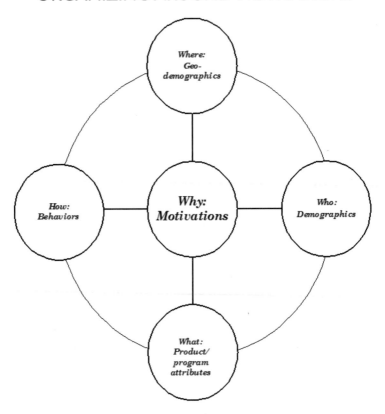

Figure 3-1: *Motivations form the hub around which other aspects can be integrated, including demographics, behaviors, and media usage.*

dicted in the *Journal of Retailing* that the mature market would become an important one. "The numbers in this age group," stated Dodge, "will continue to increase, and problems will lessen if marketers understand the nature and characteristics of the market." [2]

Diversity, not sameness

While the mature market has been and too often

continues to be viewed in massive demographic blocks, sociologists and psychologists have stressed that it is not homogeneous. This viewpoint was also influenced by gerontologists who believed mature persons differ by how they have adapted to life events.

Psychologist Erik Erikson postulated that children pass through determined psychosocial stages to adulthood. Each mature person accumulates singular life experiences that differentiate each individual. Having had fewer life experiences, five-year-olds share more similarities with their cohort than their parents and grandparents do with theirs. As sociologist Leonard Pearlin remarked, "There is not one process of aging, but many; there is not one life course, but many courses; there is no one sequence of stages, but many." [3] The many "process[es] of aging" create an incredible diversity within the mature market.

As experts in attitudinal or psychographic segmentation, we saw the need to identify and understand groups within the mature market by their attitudes toward health. Because of this need, we developed a body of work that yields not only three segmentations related to health, but also the seven critical health dimensions captured in the Morgan-Levy Health Cube.

REFERENCES

[1] Steven R. Brown. "Q Methodology and Qualitative Research." *lrz.de*. Qualitative Health Research 6.4 (1996): 561-567. Web. 15 Feb. 2011.

[2] Robert D. Dodge. "Selling the Older Consumer." *Journal of Retailing* 34.2 (1958): 73-81. Print.

[3] Leonard I. Pearlin. "Discontinuities in the study of aging." *Aging and the life course*. New York: Guilford, 1982. Print.

PART 2

Chapter 5

DIMENSIONS

Behaviors, demographics not enough

Considerable research has been done on how demographics and behaviors influence health. Far less is
known about the motivations behind the decisions we
make everyday that determine our health. As experts in
measuring motivations, we have attempted to reduce
this knowledge gap by developing the Morgan-Levy
Health Cube and its seven dimensions.

The following chapters describe the dimensions we
have researched and discovered. Each dimension represents an attitude motivating individuals to behave in
ways having either positive or negative impacts on
health. Because it is an Internet-based system, the Morgan-Levy Health Cube can be used quickly and easily.
It is, however, possible to read the following chapters
and use the information presented intuitively.

Measuring motivations

The Morgan-Levy Health Cube does not measure
behaviors or demographics. Rather it measures and reports on a person's perceptions or feelings about a
health-related issue. A high score on the Concerned

over Cost dimension, for example, does not mean someone is impoverished and unable to pay for health care. Rather it reports an individual's feelings, attitudes, or beliefs about his or her ability and willingness to pay for health care.

Moving both up and down

The seven dimensions we have discovered are a set of seven scales. After analyzing the responses of thousands of respondents, we reduced the data we gathered on health motivations to seven independent issues. The scores on each scale move both up and down the dimension. A high score on a dimension should not necessarily be viewed in a positive light. For example, a high score on the Trust in Doctors dimension indicates the individual has transferred much of the responsibility for his or her health to the doctor.

Each dimension independent

It is important to remember that these dimensions or scales are independent: each one stands on its own. A high score on the Seeks Health-related Information is not linked to a particular score on the Healthy Lifestyle dimension. Each dimension exists in its own independent silo.

What our scores mean

By completing the Morgan-Levy Health Cube questionnaire on the Internet, a score is generated on each dimension based on the individual's responses. Each score is calculated according to the statistical normal distribution, with zero representing an average based on our studies of the U.S. population 40 and older. We refer to scores one standard deviation below or above this average as "low" or "high."

35

The seven dimensions

The seven dimensions are Healthy Lifestyle, Getting a Checkup, Trust in Doctors, Self-determination, Seeks Health-related Information, Able to Understand Health Information, and Concerned over Cost. Each dimension is discussed in the following seven chapters.

Chapter contents

Every chapter begins with a brief description of the dimension and then shows the relationship between that dimension and specific behaviors and demographics. We comment only on those characteristics which correlate with the dimension at the five percent statistical significance level. We conclude each chapter with references to other studies supporting the importance of the dimension to the health of those 40 and older.

What the charts show

The data used in the charts included in each chapter contrast those persons with scores on the dimension within the highest 16 percent as compared to those with scores in the lowest 16 percent. These scores represent persons with scores above and below one standard deviation on the normal curve. Because each dimension exists on a continuum, we have had to select arbitrary high and low points on the scale.

The charts also compare those 40-to-64 in the U.S. population to those 65 and older. We believe this age breakdown provides useful comparisons between those now receiving Medicare and those who will receive it in the future.

Chapter 6

HEALTHY LIFESTYLE

DIMENSION DESCRIPTION

Those who score high on the Healthy Lifestyle dimension do not procrastinate when it comes to doing things to improve their health. They are committed to improving their health and doing whatever they can to achieve better health, including making lifestyle changes.

Those who score high on this dimension are willing to give up unhealthy behaviors in order to enjoy good health. They don't have to suffer a serious health set back in order to be motivated to make changes to achieve better health.

U.S. adults aged 40 and older who score low on the Healthy Lifestyle dimension engage in behaviors entirely opposite from those described in the above paragraphs. These behaviors range from procrastinating on making changes for better health to eating food that isn't good for them, from not exercising sufficiently to indulging in behaviors they know will have a bad effect on their health. Only a serious health crisis, if anything, motivates them to improve their health.

The Healthy Lifestyle dimension is important because moving patients or consumers up the scale to increasingly positive scores means they will be more proactive, rather than reactive, about achieving good health. By reducing unhealthy behaviors, they will increase the probability of longer and healthier lives.

RELATIONSHIPS

Demographics

A significant relationship exists between four demographic measures, age, income, number of children in the household, and gender and the Healthy Lifestyle dimension. Our research shows that as Americans age they tend to adopt attitudes reflecting increasingly healthful lifestyles. And women, in contrast to men, have higher scores on Healthy Lifestyle.

Income and the number of children in the household are negatively correlated with this dimension. The lower the income, the higher the scores on the Healthy Lifestyle dimension. We believe these relationships are most probably related to age. Because we are dealing with the 40 and older population, it follows that with increasing age both the number of children in the household and incomes decline.

Other demographics, such as years in school or marital status, do not impact on attitudes reflected in the Healthy Lifestyle dimension.

The age-related correlation we found in our data echoes research showing persons tend to postpone adopting healthful habits until their health problems become severe. And age increases the seriousness and severity of such problems. After a health-care crisis, some of those who survive go on to adopt healthier lifestyles.

While it is important to live a healthful lifestyle regardless of one's age, we would also stress the need to focus preventive programs and messages on younger persons, those in their 40s and 50s. These younger persons need to be encouraged to become proactive about living a healthful lifestyle in order to avoid chronic diseases.

Other research has shown that women are more concerned than men with preserving good health through a healthful lifestyle. A health professional who encounters a woman with a low score on the Healthy Lifestyle dimension should determine the reasons for this attitude. A man with a high score on this dimension should receive expressions of support and encouragement from his doctor or nurse.

Good health habits

Three major determinants of healthful living include normal weight in terms of body mass index (BMI), number of times one exercises at an aerobic level per week, and not smoking.

Healthy Lifestyle scores predict frequency of exercise and BMI. The higher one's score, the more frequently the person exercises each week. In addition, the higher one's score, the lower one's BMI. The score on this dimension is also predictive of smoking versus non-smoking. Those persons who are non-smokers have higher scores on the Healthy Lifestyle dimension as compared to those who are smokers.

Our data shows that the higher the score on the Healthy Lifestyle dimension, the greater the number of these three good health habits a person performs. This dimension is the only one of our seven critical dimension for which this is the case. A positive correlation exists between scores on the Healthy Lifestyle dimension and the total number of these good health habits practiced.

HEALTHY LIFESTYLE
PERCENT CURRENT SMOKERS

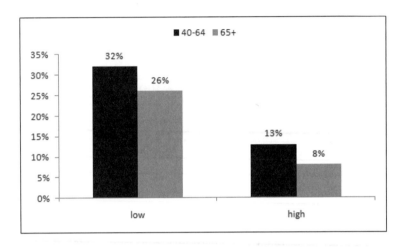

Figure 6-1: Those with low scores on the Healthy Lifestyle dimension have a far higher percentage of smokers compared to those with high scores. Regardless of their scores on this dimension, a greater percentage of those 40-to-64 are smokers as compared to those 65+ .

Use of health-care services, products

Scores on Healthy Lifestyle predict the number of prescription drugs taken daily. The higher the score on this dimension, the greater the number of prescription drugs taken.

In addition, this dimension is positively correlated to the number of doctor visits over the past year or number of days in the past two years one has been a hospital inpatient. The higher the score on the Healthy Lifestyle dimension, the greater the number of doctor visits or inpatient days generated.

40

HEALTHY LIFESTYLE
FREQUENCY OF
AEROBIC EXERCISE WEEKLY

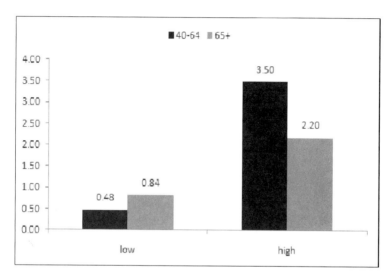

Figure 6-2: *Regardless of age, those with high scores on the Healthy Lifestyle dimension exercise more times per week at an aerobic level than those with low scores.*

Impact of disease on scores

In examining those persons with artery disease, cancer, heart disease, glaucoma or osteoporosis, we found higher scores on the Healthy Lifestyle dimension as compared to those who do not have these diseases. Conversely, those with allergies, depression, back problems, or diabetes have lower scores on this dimension.

Because a healthful lifestyle can mitigate the consequences of diabetes, it is particularly unfortunate that those with this disease have lower scores on the Healthy Lifestyle dimension.

As noted previously, higher scores on Healthy Life-

41

style are correlated with increasing age. We surmise that those who have already developed diseases included in the first group mentioned above may very well have developed attitudes placing them among the higher Healthy Lifestyle scorers, but only after developing the disease or condition. This position is supported by many studies.

It would be useful to identify those persons with either higher or lower scores on this dimension before they develop a chronic disease. Healthy persons with higher scores on the Healthy Lifestyle dimension should be encouraged to persist in their healthful behaviors.

Those with low scores who have not yet developed

HEALTHY LIFESTYLE
AVERAGE NUMBER OF CHRONIC DISEASES

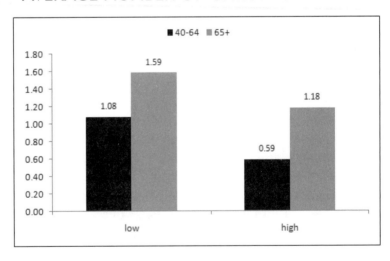

Figure 6-3: Healthy Lifestyle scores are related to both age and the number of chronic diseases one has. Older persons, as compared to younger, have higher numbers of chronic diseases. However, for both age groups, those with high Healthy Lifestyle scores have fewer chronic diseases.

a chronic disease, such as diabetes, should be encouraged to adopt more healthful attitudes. Because it reveals unhealthful attitudes, the Morgan-Levy Health Cube System can benefit persons by the early identification of attitudes that act as roadblocks to health. With insight into how negative attitudes are damaging their health, persons can decide to change or modify them, whether on their own, or with the help of a professional.

Those with low scores on the Healthy Lifestyle dimension who have already developed particular diseases must be identified and then encouraged to adopt the attitudes reflected in this dimension. Higher scores on this dimension should eventually be reflected in the healthful behaviors we have identified.

Conversely, those with high scores on the Healthy Lifestyle dimension who have developed a chronic disease should have their positive behaviors reinforced.

Multiple chronic diseases

In order to calculate each individual's number of chronic diseases, we focused on six. We grouped chronic diseases related to the heart into one category. The remaining five diseases included diabetes, depression, cancer, stroke, and upper respiratory conditions.

In calculating the total number of these chronic diseases our respondents have against their scores on the Healthy Lifestyle dimension, we found that higher scores on this dimension correlate negatively with the number of diseases reported. Specifically, those with higher scores on this dimension report fewer multiple chronic diseases.

Influencers on improving diet

Persons who reduced sodium, fat, sugar, cholesterol, and calories *on their own* have higher Healthy Lifestyle scores as compared to those who have not reduced these dietary components.

Persons who reduced the dietary factors of sodium and caffeine *on a doctor's advice* have higher scores on this dimension.

In contrast, persons who reduced sugar and calories *on a doctor's advice* have lower scores on the Healthy Lifestyle dimension.

We conclude that persons who have reduced sodium, fat, sugar, cholesterol, and calories in their diet on their own initiative are motivated to take care of themselves and live a healthful lifestyle.

Conversely, it takes a doctor's prodding to get those who don't have positive attitudes about living a healthful lifestyle to reduce sugar and calories. Without their doctor's advice, those in this group would probably not have made these beneficial changes in their diets.

Health insurance

Those who have health insurance from a major medical policy, Medicaid, or Medicare have higher scores on this dimension as contrasted to those who do not receive insurance from these sources. In contrast, those with no health insurance have lower scores on the Healthy Lifestyle dimension as contrasted to those who have any form of health insurance.

The fact that uninsured persons have lower Healthy Lifestyle scores should be very troubling to government policy makers. If the uninsured become ill, particularly because of unhealthful behaviors, they will place an additional health-care burden on a system that is already overwhelmed. Any new public healthcare initiatives will need to change both the attitudes and behaviors of those in this group.

Sources of information

Those who have paid for a health newsletter, or used a nurse, the Internet (limited to those with access), or health seminars as a source of health-related information over the past 12 months have higher scores on this dimension than those who have not used these sources.

Persons who have gotten health information over the past 12 months from advertisements on television, radio or in a magazine; as well as those who rely on a spouse (if married); other relatives or friends; or an 800 number for information on a prescription drug have lower scores contrasted to those who have not used these sources.

Persons who see the benefits of a healthful lifestyle are more apt to pay for health-related information. Those who don't believe in the importance of healthful habits are far less apt to open their wallets for such insights.

Preventive health examinations

Those who have had a mammogram (limited to females), a bone scan, or a cholesterol test within the past three years have higher scores on the Healthy Lifestyle dimension as compared to those who have not had these tests and exams.

Persons committed to a healthful lifestyle are more prone to have preventive exams to learn if they have a problem.

OTC drugs

Persons who regularly take vitamin tablets or pills, liquid vitamins, or laxatives have higher Healthy Lifestyle scores than those who do not take these over-the-counter (OTC) remedies.

45

In contrast, people who take acid blockers, antacids, antihistamines, cold medications, cough syrup, headache remedies, or who use foot-care products or skin ointments for irritation have lower scores on this dimension as compared to those who did not take such drugs.

It seems apparent that persons with more positive attitudes toward living a healthful lifestyle are more apt to take products, such as vitamins, to promote better health. Those who do not have high scores on this dimension are more likely to take or use an OTC drug or product to treat an ailment.

IMPORTANCE OF THIS DIMENSION

A chronic disease is a health condition that "limits what you can do, requires ongoing care, and lasts a year or longer."[1] Unhealthful lifestyles contribute significantly to the development of chronic diseases, such as diabetes, heart disease, and many cancers. Chronic diseases are to a large extent preventable, and yet the cost of treating such diseases threatens to overwhelm the U.S. health-care system. The 2006 Medical Expenditure Panel Survey shows that "those with chronic conditions account for 84 percent of all health care spending."[2] Patients with chronic diseases make up 82 percent of all hospital admissions, 79 percent of physicians visits, and take 92 percent of all prescriptions filled.[3]

Impact of chronic disease

Within the U.S. population, 45 percent have one or more chronic conditions.[4] Chronic diseases are, however, concentrated in those 40 and older. While more than two-thirds (68 percent) of those between 45 and 64 have one or more chronic conditions, nine out of ten

(90 percent) of those 65 and older have one or more chronic conditions.[5] The perilous financial state of the Medicare system is due in large part to the treatment of chronic diseases. The 2004 Medicare Standard Analytic File shows that "Two-thirds of Medicare spending is for beneficiaries with five or more chronic conditions."[6]

While the cost of treating chronic diseases is immense, lost economic output must also be added to its toll. The *2008 Almanac of Chronic Disease* from the Partnership to Fight Chronic Disease reports that in 2003 the cost of treating the seven most common chronic diseases, as well as lost economic output attributable to them, totaled $1.3 trillion. Indirect costs of these chronic diseases alone totaled $1 trillion. The *Almanac* projects that unless the situation changes, by 2023 the cost of both the treatment of chronic diseases and the lost economic output due to them will total $4.1 trillion.[7]

Best protection

For those 40 and older, living a healthful lifestyle is the best insurance against chronic disease and experiencing the disability, lack of independence, decrease in function, pain, and shorter lifespan that may result. Living a healthy lifestyle should be important to those in this age group not only as individuals, but also as family members, employees, and friends. Simply put, the state of one's health impacts every facet of one's life.

That mature U.S. citizens live a healthful lifestyle is also of critical importance to the country. As we have pointed out, an unhealthy lifestyle is overwhelmingly responsible for the chronic diseases that now engulf the U.S. health-care system and threaten our economy. While preventing the development of chronic disease is key to reducing health-care expenditures, it is also important to manage an existing chronic disease so that it does not worsen and require costly interventions.

Unfortunately, our work on the attitudes toward health of those 40 and older, as well as statistics on chronic disease, shows that all too many mature Americans remain uncommitted to living a healthful lifestyle.

Even a high level of education and income, as well as access to the very best health care, does not necessarily result in the practice of good health-care habits. In 2000, when more than one in three of the general U.S. population "would be classified as obese, based on objectively measured weight,"[8] a study by Dr. James Rippe, a Tufts University medical professor, found that 40 percent of 200 senior executives were obese, while 75 percent did no real exercise. These executives, with access to the very best health-insurance coverage and treatments, were not practicing the most fundamental components of a healthy lifestyle.[9]

An unhealthy lifestyle

Four behaviors mark an unhealthy lifestyle: smoking; eating an unbalanced, nutrient-poor diet; lack of sufficient physical activity; and high-risk consumption of alcohol. The Centers for Disease Control (CDC) points out in its report on "The State of Aging and Health in America 2007" that the first three behaviors "were the root causes of almost 35% of U.S. deaths in 2000."[10] The nation's chronic killers, heart disease, cancer, stroke, and diabetes, spring from these destructive behaviors.

"Adopting healthier behaviors, such as engaging in regular physical activity, eating a healthy diet, leading a tobacco free lifestyle, and getting regular health screenings . . . can dramatically reduce a person's risk for most chronic diseases, including the leading causes of death."[11] The World Health Organization (WHO) estimates that if the risk factors for chronic diseases listed above were eliminated, "at least 80% of heart disease, stroke and type 2 diabetes . . . and 40% of cancer would be prevented."[12]

Effects of smoking

According to the CDC, "Cigarette smoking continues to be the leading cause of preventable morbidity and mortality in the United States."[13] Each year, tobacco causes one in five deaths. These half million deaths include not only those who use tobacco, but also those exposed to second-hand smoke.[14]

Besides cancer, cigarette smokers also suffer from lung diseases, such as emphysema, as well as heart disease and stroke.[15] And "for every person who dies from a smoking-related disease, 20 more people suffer with at least one serious illness from smoking." Together cigarette smoking and the effects of secondhand smoke cost our country over $200 billion annually.[16]

After the 1998 Surgeon General's Report on Smoking and Health, campaigns against cigarette smoking increased. Since then, progressively more stringent laws restricting where one may smoke have been enacted, and taxes on cigarettes have increased substantially. For example, "from 2003 to 2007, there were 57 state tax increases" on cigarettes.[17] The past decade, however, has unfortunately not realized a goal set by the CDC in 2000 to reduce the percentage of smokers in the population from 23.3 percent to 12 percent by 2010.[18] In 2009, 20.6 percent of the U.S. adult population still smoked.[19]

Want to stop

When questioned, the vast majority of smokers (70

percent) say they would like to stop smoking. Each year almost half of all smokers (45 percent) actually attempt to give up cigarettes.[20] Given the extremely addictive power of cigarette smoking, it is not surprising that many of those who attempt to stop fail.

Smokers with high scores on the Healthy Lifestyle dimension reveal their interest in and commitment to living healthful lives. Those in this group appear to be a prime target for a smoking cessation program, particularly one that provides counseling and pharmacotherapy, thereby increasing the probability of success.

Obesity epidemic

A less than healthy lifestyle that includes too little exercise and too many calories often results in a condition that triggers the development of many chronic diseases: obesity. From type 2 diabetes to several types of cancer, from heart disease to stroke, obesity underlies all of these diseases.

Many researchers suggest the obesity epidemic began in the mid-1980s. In 1994 Katherine Flegal and her colleagues published findings related to the increase in obesity in the *Journal of the American Medical Association.* They found that from 1984 to 1994 "Americans had collectively gained more than a billion pounds." Writing in an editorial that accompanied the report, another researcher noted that "If this was about tuberculosis, it would be called an epidemic."[21]

In 2008 economists at RTI International estimated "The medical costs of obesity . . . to be $147 billion a year." These costs cover hospitalizations, doctor visits, and medications to treat the complications of obesity. Since 1998 obesity rates have risen 37 percent, and the costs to treat it have almost doubled. On an annual basis, obese persons "spent $1,429 more on medical care than normal weight people," costs borne by public and private insurers, as well as by employers and the patients themselves. This study finds that from 1998 to 2008 the aggregated annual "medical burden of obesity . . . increased from 6.5 percent to 9.1 percent of annual medical spending."[22]

The future is fat

While two-thirds of the mature population today is considered to be either overweight or obese as determined by their body-mass index, this percentage is projected to increase dramatically in the years ahead.

Reporting on a survey entitled "F as in Fat: How Obesity Policies are Failing America" from the Trust for America's Health and the Robert Wood Johnson Foundation, a *Bloomberg Businessweek* reporter notes the baby boom generation, now crossing over into retirement, is "the fattest cohort yet." In every state, "the 55-to-64 age group has a higher rate of obesity than people over 65, an ominous sign for Medicare."[23]

Long lives, sick lives

Obesity and the chronic diseases it brings will result in long, although sicker, lives. Researchers point out that "overweight people tend to live as long as the thin, but with far more chronic diseases that are costly to treat." Dr. James S. Marks, a senior vice president at the Robert Wood Johnson Foundation, states that "There is a huge wave of obese adults coming that will bankrupt us as a nation unless we get this under control now."[24]

Into denial

Unfortunately, many of those who are overweight or obese deny their condition. A McClatchy-Ipsos poll conducted in 2009 found that most Americans deny they have a serious weight problem. This position is contradicted by government data collected over the past 20 years showing a staggering increase in obesity in the United States. The poll found that almost half (49 percent) of the respondents said that "it [obesity] was no problem at all." Two-thirds of those surveyed felt they were at a healthy weight, while just four percent said they were very overweight. These positions fly in the face of government data showing that only one state, Colorado, has an obesity rate of 20 percent, the lowest in the U.S.[25]

Fat accepted

Recent studies show that fewer people who are overweight or obese are committed to doing something about it. The NPD Group's Annual Report on Eating Patterns in America presents survey results showing that "The number of people on a diet—26 percent of all women in the United States and 16 percent of men for the year ending February 2008—is the lowest it has been in more than two decades . . . " In 1990, the same report found 39 percent of women and 29 percent of men were dieting.

Besides not trying to lose weight, more Americans don't consider their additional pounds to be unattractive. "In 1985, 55 percent of those surveyed 'completely agreed' with the statement, 'People who are not overweight look a lot more attractive.' Today only 25 percent completely agree with it."[26]

A study reported in the journal *Economic Inquiry* found that " . . . weight norms may change and are not set standards based on beauty or medical ideals." As more people in the United States carry around a spare tire, being overweight or obese has become increasingly socially acceptable. This study found that not only has women's actual weight edged up, but the perceived ideal weight has also increased.[27]

Prevention underfunded

According to the previously mentioned McClatchy-Ipsos survey, 75 percent of Americans believe that "the most effective way to combat obesity is through education about the importance of exercise and a healthy diet . . ."[28] But as the number of overweight and obese Americans increases, the U.S. spends little on preventive efforts of any type. Of the $7,681 spent on U.S. health care per resident in 2008, three percent went to government public health expenditures.[29] In our opinion, as well as others, such efforts are insufficient.

New perspective needed

In contrast, the World Health Organization (WHO) believes that "To conquer obesity will . . . require a complete new awareness, the re-education of the great mass of consumers . . ." The WHO believes this re-education "seems a distant prospect."[30] However distant the prospect, solving the crisis in healthy lifestyles is critical. As Thomas Kottke and Nicolaas P. Pronk, both of HealthPartners, a Minnesota-based health maintenance organization (HMO), point out in an editorial, "The evidence indicates the crisis in health care can be solved only if the crisis in healthy lifestyles is solved, too."[31]

Behaviors, motivations linked

While there is agreement that something must be done to avoid chronic diseases and to control their worsening, the focus of current strategies to improve the lifestyles of those 40 and older is largely on behaviors. In contrast, we have developed a deep understand-

53

ing of the health-related motivations of this population. In this chapter's previous section we linked the motivational perspective expressed in our key Healthy Lifestyle dimension to actual behaviors from our data.

These linkages show that there is indeed a statistically significant relationship between the motivation to live a healthful lifestyle expressed in high scores on our Healthy Lifestyle dimension and behaviors that support it. The reverse, unfortunately, is also evident in the case of low scores on this dimension. Beyond the significant relationships between motivations and behaviors related to the Healthy Lifestyle dimension, we have in our chapter on validity demonstrated the predictive value of our system.

REFERENCES

[1] Gerard Anderson, ed. "Chronic Conditions: Making the Case for Ongoing Care." *fightchronicdisease.org*. Pres. Johns Hopkins Bloomberg School of Public Health and the Robert Wood Johnson Foundation, Feb. 2010. Web. 1 June 2010.

[2] Gerard Anderson, ed.

[3] Gerard Anderson, ed.

[4] "The Growing Crisis of Chronic Disease in the United States." *fightchronicdisease.org*. The Partnership to Fight Chronic Disease. Web. 1 June 2010.

[5] Gerard Anderson, ed.

[6] Gerard Anderson, ed.

[7] "The Almanac of Chronic Disease." *fightchronicdisease.org*. The Partnership to Fight Chronic Disease. Web. 1 June 2010.

[8] R. Sturm. "Increases in morbid obesity in the USA: 2000 to 2005." *ncbi.nlm.nih.gov*. Public Health. 30 March 2007. Web. 30 July 2011.

[9] Walter Gaman. "Executive Health a Top Priority for Stock Holders." *corporatewellnessmagazine.com*. 1 Jan. 2011. Web. 30 July 2011.

[10] Centers for Disease Control and Prevention. "The State of Aging and Health in America 2007." *cdc.gov*. Web. 1 June 2010.

[11] "The State of Aging and Health in America 2007."

[12] "Ten facts about chronic disease." *who.int*. World Health Organization. Web. 1 June 2010.

[13] Centers for Disease Control and Prevention. "Vital Signs: Current Cigarette Smoking Among Adults Aged > 18 Years—United States, 2009." *cdc.gov*. Web. 18 Nov. 2010.

[14] Centers for Disease Control and Prevention. "Fast Facts: Tobacco use is the leading preventable cause of death." *cdc.gov*. Web. 29 Nov. 2010.

[15] Centers for Disease Control and Prevention. "Fast Facts: Tobacco use leads to disease and disability." *cdc.gov*. Web. Nov. 2010.

[16] Centers for Disease Control and Prevention. "Fast Facts: Tobacco use costs the United States billions of dollars each year." *cdc.gov*. Web. 29 Nov. 2010.

[17]Shaila Dewan. "States Look to Tobacco to Balance the Budget." *nytimes.com.* New York Times, 20 March 2009. Web. 18 Nov. 2010.

[18] Centers for Disease Control and Prevention. "Cigarette Smoking Among Adults—United States, 2000." *cdc.gov.* Web. 18 Nov. 2010.

[19] Centers for Disease Control and Prevention. "Fast Facts: Tobacco Use in the United States." *cdc.gov.* Web. 29 Nov. 2010.

[20] Centers for Disease Control and Prevention. "Fast Facts: Many adult smokers want or try to quit smoking." *cdc.gov.* Web. 29 Nov. 2010.

[21] Elizabeth Kolbert. "XXXL Why are we so fat?" *newyorker.com.* New Yorker, 20 July 2009. Web. 1 June 2010.

[22] Sarah Avery. "Obesity costs billions, economists say." *newsobserver.com.* The News & Observer, 27 July 2009. Web. 1 June 2010.

[23] Catherine Arnst. "Fat in the USA: Obesity is Rising." *businessweek.com.* Bloomberg BusinessWeek, 1 July 2009. Web. 1 June 2010.

[24] Arnst.

[25] William Douglas. "Poll: Americans claim that they're not so fat." *mcclatchydc.com.* McClatchy Newspapers, 6 Aug. 2009. Web. 1 June 2010.

[26] Beth Teitell. "Interest in dieting slims down; More accepting the extra pounds." *boston.com.* Boston Globe, 21 Sept. 2008. Web. 1 June 2010.

[27] "Americans see fat as normal as weights rise: study," *reuters.com*. Reuters Life!, 7 Aug. 2007. Web. 2 June 2010.

[28] Douglas.

[29] "U.S. Health Care Costs." *kaiseredu.org*. The Henry J. Kaiser Family Foundation. Web. 27 May 2010.

[30] Kolbert.

[31] Thomas Kottke and Nicolaas P. Pronk. "Health care reform? Don't forget the simple things that matter most." *St. Paul Pioneer Press* 11 Jan. 2009, B11. Print.

Chapter 7

GETTING A CHECKUP

DIMENSION DESCRIPTION

High scorers on this dimension are convinced of the benefits of an annual checkup and are open to doctor visits. They have a methodical approach to scheduling checkups, which include having their eyesight and hearing checked by specialists.

On the other hand, low scorers on this dimension lack a commitment to getting regular checkups. Even if a specialist conducts specific tests and exams, low scorers on this dimension don't consider them important.

This dimension establishes a person's willingness to be examined by a doctor, whether on a regular basis or as needed. In addition, it predicts whether or not those who already have a chronic disease will schedule regular follow-up visits with their doctors. We know that if many diseases are either caught early or managed successfully, which is more likely with regular checkups, the possibility for cost savings and positive outcomes is greatly increased.

RELATIONSHIPS

Demographics

Within those 40 and older in the U.S. population, scores on the Getting a Checkup dimension correlate positively with increasing age, as well as incomes. Persons who are married also have higher scores on the Getting a Checkup dimension.

Those who are older have a stronger belief in the importance of getting a checkup or visiting their doctor. This makes sense: the probability of illness increases with age. And increasing health problems result in a greater number of doctor visits. Those with higher incomes can better afford health insurance premiums, as well as co-payments. Those who are married may very well be concerned with maintaining the health of their significant other.

In contrast, the number of children in the home correlates negatively with this dimension. The greater the number of children living in the home, the lower the score on the Getting a Checkup dimension. This relationship is probably a function of age.

Good health habits

There are no significant relationships between the attitudinal dimension of Getting a Checkup and three major determinants of a healthful lifestyle: a normal weight in terms of BMI, the number of times one exercises at an aerobic level weekly, and not smoking.

Impact of disease on scores

Persons with allergies, artery disease, arthritis, cancer, congestive heart failure, heart disease, depression, diabetes, high blood pressure, osteoporosis, or back problems have higher scores on the Getting a Checkup dimension. Most of these diseases require physician monitoring and, therefore, the need for checkups or doctor visits.

GETTING A CHECKUP
AVERAGE NUMBER OF CHRONIC DISEASES

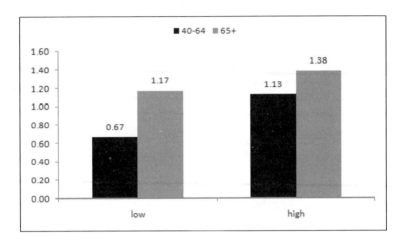

Figure 7-1: *Persons with high scores on this dimension have more chronic diseases than those with low scores. Those with high scores who are 40-to-64 have as many chronic diseases as those with low scores who are older.*

Those who suffer from chronic migraines have significantly lower scores on the Getting a Checkup dimension.

Persons with chronic, life-threatening diseases with lower scores on this dimension who don't see their doctor when necessary should be told they are indulging in risky behavior.

Multiple chronic diseases

Using a group of six chronic diseases, we examined

the actual number of chronic diseases our respondents have against their scores on the Getting a Checkup dimension. We found that higher scores on this dimension correlate positively with the number of chronic diseases each person reported. Specifically, those with higher scores on this dimension have a greater number of the chronic diseases on which our analysis was based.

Influencers on improving diet

Persons who have reduced sodium, fat, sugar, and calories *on a doctor's advice* have higher scores on this dimension. Those who have reduced cholesterol whether *on a doctor's advice* or *on their own* also have higher scores on the Getting a Checkup dimension.

Persons who reduced fat in their diet *on their own* have lower scores on this dimension.

Use of health-related services, products

As one would expect, the higher the score on this dimension, the greater the number of all of the following: number of doctor visits annually, prescription drugs taken on a daily basis, as well as the number of both in- and outpatient days spent in a hospital over the past two years.

Health insurance

It is not surprising that persons with no health insurance have lower scores on the Getting a Checkup dimension as contrasted to those who have health insurance coverage. The former group's lack of access has obviously influenced their attitudes about the importance of visiting a doctor. The uninsured deal with the reality that without health insurance it is difficult, if not impossible, to get necessary medical care.

Patients with lower scores on this dimension with a serious disease and who have health insurance need to be advised to get the checkups provided by their health plans. If they do not do so, they risk greater health problems and, ultimately, higher health-care costs.

GETTING A CHECKUP
AVERAGE NUMBER OF RX TAKEN DAILY

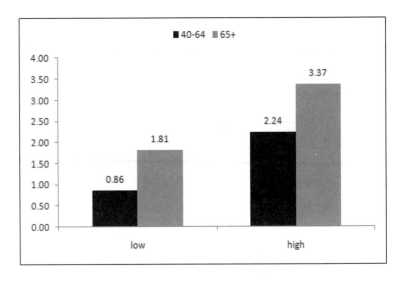

Figure 7-2: Those with high scores on the Getting a Checkup dimension take more prescription drugs daily as compared to those with low scores. Older persons take more prescription drugs daily than those who are younger.

Persons receiving health-care coverage from a managed care organization, a major medical health insurance policy, the Veterans Administration (VA), or Medicare have higher scores on the Getting a Checkup dimension as compared to those who do not get health insurance from these sources.

Sources of information

Persons who received health-related information from doctors, nurses, pharmacists, employer (if employed), newspapers, non-health-related magazines, or health organizations over the past 12 months have higher scores on the Getting a Checkup dimension as compared to those who did not use these sources of information.

GETTING A CHECKUP
DOCTOR VISITS ANNUALLY

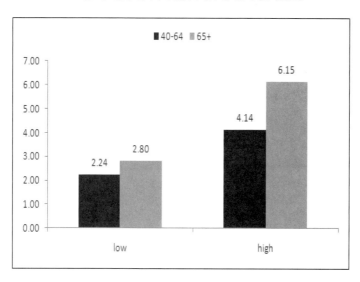

Figure 7-3: Those with high scores on this dimension see the doctor more times per year than those with low scores. It is interesting to note that those 40-to-64 with high scores make more doctor visits than those with low scores in the older age group.

Those who have received health-related information over the past 12 months from advertisements on television, radio, or in a magazine; a spouse (if married); or books are more likely to have lower scores on the Getting a Checkup dimension.

It is evident that for this group health-related information is provided by informal, accessible, and low- or no-cost sources. It is critical that governments, health-promotion organizations, such as the American Diabetes Association, and others communicate with increasing effectiveness with them.

Preventive health examinations

Those who have had each of the six tests we track within the last three years have higher scores on the Getting a Checkup dimension as compared to those who have not had these tests. These preventive health exams include the following: a mammogram and Pap test (limited to women), as well as a bone scan, hemoglobin A1c, and cholesterol and blood pressure evaluations.

OTC drugs

Regular users of the following OTC products have higher scores on this dimension as compared to those who do not use them: foot care, hair growth, skin lotions for dry skin, skin ointments for pain, or vitamins, whether tablets or pills, Those who take no OTC drugs regularly are more apt to have lower scores on the Getting a Checkup dimension.

IMPORTANCE OF THIS DIMENSION

Value of checkups, doctor visits

Checkups, health exams, and doctor visits are necessary in order to prevent, diagnose, and treat disease. According to the Centers for Disease Control (CDC),

"Regular health exams and tests can help . . . find problems before they start. They also can help find problems early, when . . . chances for treatment and cure are better. . ."[1] The CDC finds that ". . . getting the right health services, screenings, and treatments . . ." increases the probability that one will lead "a longer, healthier life."[2]

While the U.S. Preventive Services Task Force determined ten years ago that the routine physical is unnecessary for "healthy, asymptomatic persons,"[3] it also agreed that this population should still have certain tests and exams periodically. Included within this group are exams such as colorectal screenings and blood pressure tests.

Two diseases illustrate need

The need for checkups or doctor visits is exemplified by two conditions or diseases: high blood pressure and diabetes. Posing serious problems to public health, these two diseases are all too often either not prevented, remain undiagnosed, or are insufficiently controlled.

In the U.S. today 74.5 million people or an estimated one in three adults 20 and older have high blood pressure.[4] In the Western world a person "has a greater than 90% lifetime risk of developing high blood pressure or hypertension."[5] Although high blood pressure is easily diagnosed with a simple and inexpensive test at a doctor's office, approximately 25 percent of those with this condition are unaware they have it.

Dealing with an epidemic

Among those 20 and older in the U.S. population with high blood pressure, 78.3 percent have either not been diagnosed with high blood pressure or, if diagnosed and under treatment, do not have their high blood pressure under control.[6] A group of experts on an Institute of Medicine panel determined that "Out-of-control and undiagnosed hypertension is at epidemic proportions in the United States."[7]

Controlling high blood pressure, an unseen and often unfelt disease, depends on patient compliance. Offering diagnosis, education, prescription medications, support, and monitoring, doctor visits play a critical role in the control of high blood pressure. In 2006 two out of every three U.S. patients had their blood pressure checked when they saw their doctor.[8] During that year, Americans visited their doctors "more than 40 million times to treat their high blood pressure."[9]

Impact of doctor visits

The frequency of these doctor visits, as well as the number of times a patient is told he or she has high blood pressure, appear key to its control. For example, a study conducted by the CDC found that 19.4 percent of the respondents had been told two or more times they had high blood pressure.[10] Of this group, roughly two out of three had changed their eating habits, were exercising, took hypertensive medication, and had also reduced or eliminated salt.

In a separate study of diabetics with high blood pressure, patients who saw their doctor monthly took an average of 1.5 months to achieve normal blood pressure levels. In contrast, "patients who waited longer between visits took an average of 12.2 months for their readings to return to normal." Those who saw their doctor every two weeks had the best results of all.[11]

A leading cause of death

The value of diagnosing and controlling hypertension is easily seen. Hypertension, or high blood pressure, is the second leading cause of death in the U.S.[12]

Besides the number of deaths attributable to high blood pressure, a report from the World Health Organization (WHO) found hypertension "responsible for 3.8% of years of life lost due to premature death plus years of healthy life lost due to illness and disability . . . ."[13] In 2006 "for every 1000 US workers, 4.5 weeks of work were lost due to an episode of hypertension."[14]

As with hypertension, diabetes too remains a disease that too often escapes diagnosis. A report published in *Population Health Management* suggests that "about 6.3 million adults—about a fourth of the people in the U.S. with diabetes—have the disease but haven't been diagnosed."[15]

Massive financial burden

According to the study, undiagnosed diabetics are responsible for "an estimated $18 billion in health care costs annually . . . ."[16] These increased health-care costs begin to mount "at least eight years before diagnosis" and cover such things as "ambulatory visits, emergency room visits, and hospital inpatient days . . . ."[17] Because diabetes impacts virtually every part of the body, medical costs for undiagnosed diabetes include "$2.3 billion for cardiovascular disease . . . [and] $443 million for kidney problems."[18]

Recent CDC data show that "nearly half of the U.S. population has at least one of three diagnosed or undiagnosed chronic conditions—high blood pressure, high cholesterol, or diabetes . . . . CDC researchers also found that 15 percent of adults also had one or more of these conditions undiagnosed."[19]

Impact of failed appointments

All three of these conditions are known to increase the risk for cardiovascular disease, the primary cause of death in the U.S. The importance of physician visits—

and the tests and examinations which are often included in those visits—cannot be contested. But some persons avoid scheduling a physician visit or even when they do, they don't keep it. All too many patients do not return to their doctors for the follow-up care they need.

The failure to show up for a scheduled appointment with a doctor ranges from 12 percent to 42 percent.[20] The Sibley Heart Center at Children's Healthcare of Atlanta, which handles 30,000 outpatient appointments annually, experienced a "16.7% same-day cancellation and no-show rate."[21]

While no-shows for a medical appointment are a significant problem in health-care delivery, recent research reveals missed specialist referrals as another. A study on patients 65 and older showed that "only 71% were ever scheduled for a needed follow-up appointment." Of that 71 percent only 70 percent were actually seen by the specialist, "meaning that just 50% received the treatment that their primary-care doctor intended them to have." This high percentage led the researchers to call "missed specialist referrals the most frequent error in medicine."[22]

A disruption in care

Because failed or never scheduled appointments disrupt a patient's continuity of care, their consequences can be immense. In the case of diabetics, for example, researchers found that patients who fail appointments "have significantly more risk factors and complications than those who keep their appointments."[23] By missing an appointment—or never scheduling one in the first place—patients remain undiagnosed, uninformed, and lacking support in any treatment. Worse health-care outcomes are the almost inevitable result.

Besides the less than optimal care received by a patient who avoids making and keeping a health-care appointment, there is also the cost to the health-care system of such missed appointments or no shows. Excluding emergency room care and care provided by the federal government, government data shows that 9.7 million doctor visits were provided between 2001 and 2002 to the U.S. population.[24] It is true that estimates for the percentage of doctor visits which become same-day cancellations or no shows varies widely, ranging from 5 to 42 percent. We believe that 10 percent is a conservative and defensible percentage for lost doctor visits.

Again taking a conservative position on the percent of lost visits, we estimate the cost of no-shows or last minute cancellations at $1.5 billion annually. In 2004, the "average expense for an office-based physician visit was $155."[25] One study has estimated that clinics lose from "3-14% of total out patient income in the United States" from same-day cancellations or no shows.[26] We conclude that such cancellations are both a significant waste of resources and a major threat to both patient health and clinic revenues.

The points made above underscore the importance of the Getting a Checkup dimension. Measuring the patient's own attitudes toward getting a checkup or making a doctor's appointment, this dimension is an important measure of a willingness to participate in one's own health care.

REFERENCES

[1] "Regular Check-Ups Are Important." Department of Health and Human Services, Centers for Disease Control and Prevention. *cdc.gov.* Web. 22 June 2010.

[2] "Regular Check-Ups Are Important."

[3] Sally Farhat. "The Annual Physical: Do You Really Need That Yearly Checkup?" *msn.com*. MSN Health & Fitness. Web. 22 June 2010.

[4] "High Blood Pressure Statistics." American Heart Association. *americanheart.org*. Web. 25 Oct. 2010.

[5] "Blood pressure cases 'to top 1bn.'" *newsvote.bbc.co.uk*. BBC News. Web. 22 June 2010.

[6] American Heart Association. "Heart Disease and Stroke Statistics—2010 update." *circ.ahajournals.org*. Web. 25 Oct. 2010.

[7] Brenda Wilson. "Hypertension: A Growing but Often Hidden Problem." *npr.org*. NPR, *Morning Edition*. Web. 29 March 2010.

[8] Centers for Disease Control and Prevention. "High Blood Pressure Facts." *cdc.gov*. Web. 22 Oct. 2010.

[9] "High Blood Pressure Facts."

[10] "Frequent Doctor Visits Help Diabetics Control Blood Pressure." *medicinenet.com*. HealthDayNews, May 24, 2010. Web. 23 Oct. 2010.

[11] "Frequent Doctor Visits Help Diabetics Control Blood Pressure."

[12] Wilson.

[13] Linda Brookes Good. "Hypertension Highlights: Blood Pressure Targets, Global Risk Factors, and Diabetes—the Latest Data Are Not Encouraging," *medscape.com*. Medscape Cardiology. Web. 24 June 2010.

[14] Brookes Good.

[15] Linda Brookes. "The Epidemiology of Hyptertension: Latest Data and Statistics: New Report Documents Economic Impact of Hypertension in the United States." *medscape.com*. WebMD Professional. Web. 24 June 2010.

[16] Bill Hendrick, "Costs Are High From Undiagnosed Diabetes," *webmd.com*. WebMD Health News. Web. 22 June 2010.

[17] Hendrick.

[18] Hendrick.

[19] Katrina Woznicki. "Many in U.S. Have at Least 1 Heart Risk Factor." *medicinenet.com*. WebMD Health News. Web. 22 June 2010.

[20] Vernon J. Lee, et al. "Predictors of failed attendances in a multi-specialty outpatient centre using electronic databases." *nlm.nih.gov*. BMC Health Services Research 5.51 (2005). Web. 28 June 2010.

[21] Anya Martin. "Preventing missed appointments with specialists." *marketwatch.com*. MarketWatch, 22 April 2010. Web. 29 June 2010.

[22] Martin.

[23] S. J. Griffin. "Lost to follow-up: the problem of defaulters from diabetes clinics." *ncbi.nlm.nih.gov.* Diabetic Medicine S14-24 (1998). Web. 29 June 2010.

[24] Centers for Disease Control and Prevention, Feb. 2006. "Ambulatory Care Visits to Physician Offices, Hospital Out-patient Departments, and Emergency Departments: United States, 2001-02." *cdc.gov.* Web. 30 June 2010.

[25] Steven R. Machlin and Kelly Carper. "Expenses for Office-Based Visits by Specialty, 2004." *ahrq.gov.* Agency for Healthcare Research and Quality, March 2007. Web. 25 May 2011.

[26] Lee, et al.

Chapter 8

TRUST IN DOCTORS

DIMENSION DESCRIPTION

Those who score high on this dimension believe their doctors care about them. The high scorers' feeling of having a human connection with their doctor supports a belief that their doctor knows best when treating health problems.

High scorers believe following their doctor's instructions is the best way to enjoy good health, and they follow these instructions completely. Faith in their doctors is, then, linked to a high level of compliance with a physician's recommendations and instructions.

Those who score low on this dimension feel their doctors don't care about them. Believing their doctors do not appreciate them as persons, low scorers don't trust or rely on what their doctors advise them to do. Low scorers on this dimension aren't secure in the knowledge that a caring doctor gives them reliable advice. These low scorers are not motivated to be compliant.

Identifying a patient's position on this dimension will help doctors develop greater rapport with their patients. In addition, this increased rapport and a more open relationship should generate greater compliance.

RELATIONSHIPS

Demographics

Within the 40 and older population, statistically significant relationships exists between the Trust in Doctors dimension and all the demographic variables in our analysis.

Our data shows that the older the American, the higher the score on the Trust in Doctors dimension. Higher scores on this dimension are also given by males, in contrast to females, and those who are married, as opposed to those who are single.

This dimension is negatively correlated with income, education, and the number of children in the household. Those with higher incomes, higher levels of education, or a greater number of children in the household have lower scores on a feeling or belief that doctors should be trusted and their advice followed.

Good health habits

Taken individually, whether someone smokes or not or has a normal BMI or not, is not related to his or her score on the Trust in Doctors dimension.

In contrast, a negative correlation exists between the number of times one exercises at an aerobic level weekly and this dimension. Those who have higher scores on the Trust in Doctors dimension exercise fewer times per week.

We found a negative correlation between the three major determinants of a healthful lifestyle and the attitudinal dimension of Trust in Doctors. Those with higher Trust in Doctors dimension scores exhibit lower numbers of these three good health habits.

We see, then, that a high level of trust in one's doctor does not result in a commitment to a regular exercise program, the cessation of smoking, or to a lower

BMI. Patients with higher scores on this dimension may believe their doctor will save them from their less than healthful behaviors.

TRUST IN DOCTORS
FREQUENCY OF
AEROBIC EXERCISE WEEKLY

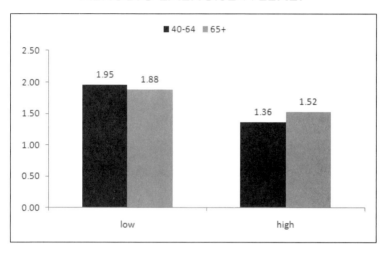

Figure 8-1: Regardless of age group, those with low scores on this dimension exercise more frequently than those with high scores.

Use of health-related services, products

Trust in Doctors dimension scores correlate positively with the number of prescription drugs taken daily, as well as the number of days spent hospitalized over the past two years. Thus, the more patients trust their doctors, the more likely they are to take a greater number of prescription drugs and spend more days hospitalized as an inpatient. In addition, the higher the scores on the Trust in Doctors dimension the greater the number of doctor visits per year.

Since doctors write prescriptions and determine

75

hospital admissions, this relationship is understandable. Both of these behaviors are directly linked to sicker patients. And, as we note below, persons with one or more very serious illnesses have significantly higher scores on the Trust in Doctors dimension.

TRUST IN DOCTORS
AVERAGE NUMBER OF HOSPITAL
INPATIENT DAYS PAST TWO YEARS

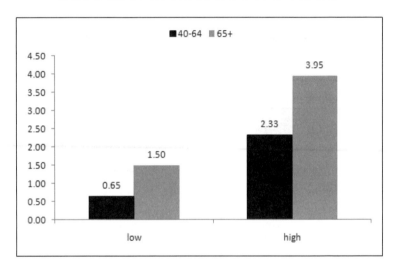

Figure 8-2: Those with high scores on this dimension have spent more days as inpatients over the last two years as compared to those with low scores. We find that those 40-to-64 with high scores have spent more hospital days as inpatients as compared to those older with low scores.

Impact of disease on scores

Those who have artery disease, cancer, heart disease, congestive heart failure, diabetes, glaucoma or high blood pressure have higher scores on the Trust in Doctors dimension.

On the other hand, those who have allergies, chronic migraines, depression, osteoporosis, back problems, or sinus problems have lower scores on this dimension.

The diseases prevalent among higher scorers are serious ones. In most cases, they are life-threatening. We assume those with these diseases would necessarily have to have a higher level of trust in their doctors.

TRUST IN DOCTORS
AVERAGE NUMBER OF RX TAKEN DAILY

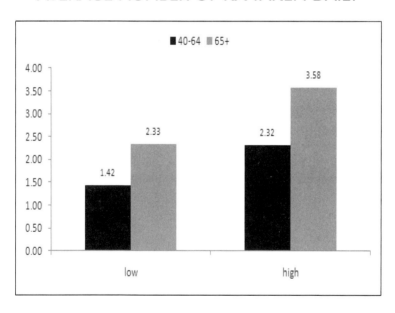

Figure 8-3: Those 65+ take more prescription drugs daily than those 40-to-64. However, within both age groups, those with high scores on this dimension take a greater number of prescription drugs daily than those with low scores.

Multiple chronic diseases

After totaling each individual's actual number of

chronic diseases from a group of six, including cancer, cardiovascular disease, stroke, upper respiratory disease, depression, and diabetes, we then measured the total number of diseases against our respondent's scores on the Trust in Doctors dimension.

We found that scores on this dimension do not correlate with the number of diseases reported. Specifically, scores on this dimension do not predict the number of chronic diseases from this group of diseases.

Influencers on improving diet

Those who have reduced sodium, fat, sugar, cholesterol, and calories *on a doctor's advice* have higher scores on the Trust in Doctors dimension. Those who reduced cholesterol *on their own* have lower scores on this dimension.

We conclude that many patients with higher scores on this dimension can be persuaded to lower their intake of a potentially damaging food component, such as sodium, if their doctor tells them to do so. This group, however, will not take such action on its own initiative.

Those with lower scores on this dimension will most likely only reduce cholesterol on their own. They will do so not because of their doctor's advice, but possibly because of some other influence, such as the popular media or a family member.

Health insurance

Six sources of health insurance are included in our research. Higher scores on the Trust in Doctors dimension are seen in two types of health insurance. Persons who have a major medical policy or Medicare have higher scores on this dimension than those who do not.

Those who are insured by a managed-care organization are more likely to have lower scores on this dimension.

This outcome should be troubling to providers of this form of health insurance. It may be that those who are 40 and older and enrolled in managed care believe their doctors make health-care decisions with one eye on the bottom line. These patients may have concluded that doctors working under managed care have less freedom to order services. These types of perceptions may lead to an erosion of trust.

Sources of information

In our questionnaires we have asked about 21 sources of health information used in the past 12 months, ranging from doctors to newspaper articles, the government to employers.

Persons who use paid health newsletters, doctors, nurses, pharmacists, their spouse (among those who are married), or those who use videotapes have higher scores on the Trust in Doctors dimension in contrast to those who do not use these sources. Those who use non-health-related magazines, newspapers, books, the Internet (limited to those with access), relatives and friends, employer (if employed), or government publications have lower scores on this dimension in contrast to those who don't use them.

It is possible that some of these findings are influenced by demographics. We have already noted that lower scores on this dimension are seen among those who are more educated and younger. More likely users of the Internet are found among both of these demographic groups. Furthermore, older persons, who typically have a greater number of health concerns, have more frequent contact with health professionals.

Preventive health examinations

We found no relationship between four of the six preventive health tests and examinations we track and those with either higher or lower scores on the Trust in Doctors dimension. However, those who have had a hemoglobin A1c test in the past three years have significantly higher scores on this dimension. On the other hand, those who have had their blood pressure tested over that time period have lower scores on this dimension.

OTC drugs

Persons who use antacids, cold medications, cough syrups, laxatives, skin ointments for irritation or sleeping pills have higher scores on this dimension as compared to those who do not use such products. A doctor's suggestion may influence the increased tendency to take such OTC remedies.

In contrast, those who take no OTC drugs on a regular basis have lower scores on the Trust in Doctors dimension. Persons who take or use OTC remedies for hair growth, diet pills, energy boosters, herbal medications, memory enhancers, potency enhancers, or skin ointments for pain also have lower scores as compared to those who do not use these products. Used for occasional acute problems or enhancements, these remedies are probably used without a doctor's suggestion.

IMPORTANCE OF THIS DIMENSION

At a 2003 symposium sponsored by Johns Hopkins entitled "Defining the Patient-Physician Relationship for the 21st Century," over two hundred medical professionals and consumers met to define this critical relationship.

The group concluded that "The fundamental inter-action in health care is the one between patient and physician. That fact, moreover, is likely to remain true for the foreseeable future. . . . the patient-physician re-lationship is the touchstone to which the entire system must align. . . ." In defining the patient-physician rela-tionship, participants in the symposium began "with only one assumption": this all-important relationship should be "rooted in mutual trust and respect . . . ."

Relationship supports health

Those attending the symposium stressed that if this rela-tionship functions optimally, "the physician-patient relation-ship not only gives patients access to health care but also can promote healing." They noted that ". . . mounting evidence demonstrates that the effectiveness of the patient-physician relationship directly relates to health outcomes."[1]

For example, "A smoker's chances of quitting success-fully . . . rise substantially if a doctor gets involved. Studies have shown that just a three-minute conversation between patient and doctor can increase chances of success by 30%."[2]

Two recent studies "show that whether patients trust a doctor strongly influences whether they take their medica-tion."[3] And yet another study found that "patients with higher trust in their physician were significantly more likely to report engaging in eight recommended health behaviors, including exercise, smoking cessation, and safe sexual prac-tices."[4]

In reviewing "21 randomized controlled trials and ana-lytic studies on the effects of physician-patient communica-tion on patient health outcomes, the quality of communica-tion in both history taking and discussion of the management plan was found to be associated with health outcomes. Better doctor patient communication was shown to be associated with better emotional and physical health, higher symptom resolution, and better control of chronic diseases that included better blood pressure, blood glucose and pain control."[5]

An erosion of trust

Recent articles suggest, however, that the patient-physician relationship has deteriorated over the past decades. "A growing chorus of discontent suggests that the once-revered doctor-patient relationship is on the rocks."[6] One example of this discontent is seen in the fact that "About one in four patients feel that their physicians sometimes expose them to unnecessary risk, according to data from a Johns Hopkins study published . . . in the journal *Medicine*."[7]

Doctors say they are not surprised at the negative relationship between patients and physicians. "It's been striking to me . . . how unhappy patients are and, frankly, how mistreated patients are," said Dr. Sandeep Jauhar, director of the heart failure program at Long Island Jewish Medical Center and an occasional contributor to *Science Times*.[8]

The patient-physician relationship, which some believe is currently in a less than optimal state, will continue to be shaped and reshaped in the 21st century by complex economic and social forces. We have noted that trust between patient and physician forms the very foundation of health care and that the quality of the patient-physician relationship influences health outcomes: ". . . the absence or presence of trust in patient-provider relations can have life-changing consequences. A person who trusts a provider is more likely to seek care, comply with treatment recommendations, and return for follow-up care than a person who has little trust in a specific provider . . ."[9]

Given the importance of the doctor-patient relationship, we believe it is critical to systematically measure the patient's relationship with doctors as indicated by our Trust in Doctors dimension.

REFERENCES

[1] "Defining the Patient-Physician Relationship for the 21st Century." *cardiophonics.com*. 3rd Annual Disease Management Outcomes Summit. American Healthways and Johns Hopkins. Phoenix, Arizona. 30 Oct. 2003. Web. 17 July 2010.

[2] Vanessa Fuhrmans. "Case Grows to Cover Quitting." *online.wsj.com*. Wall Street Journal, 26 April 2005. Web. 17 July 2010.

[3] Tara Parker-Pope. "Doctor and Patient, Now at Odds." *nytimes.com*. New York Times, 29 July 2008. Web. 15 July 2010.

[4] David H. Thom, et al. "Measuring Patients' Trust in Physicians When Assessing Quality of Care." *healthaffairs.org*. Health Affairs 23.4 (2004): 124-132. Web. 15 July 2010.

[5] Samuel Y.S. Wong and Albert Lee. "Communication Skills and the Doctor Patient Relationship." *fmshk.com.hk*. Medical Bulletin 2.3 (2006): 7-9. Web. 23 June 2010.

[6] Parker-Pope.

[7] Parker-Pope.

[8] Parker-Pope.

[9] Thom, et al.

Chapter 9

SELF-DETERMINATION

DIMENSION DESCRIPTION

Those who score high on this dimension have retained the locus of control for their health care. They are convinced they themselves are in charge of their health, not their doctors. High scorers believe they are healthy and rarely get sick.

They equate taking a prescription drug to giving up control over their health. In an attempt to avoid taking such drugs, those who score high on this dimension commit themselves to exercise and a healthy lifestyle. They will try other options before taking a prescription drug.

Conversely, low scorers on this dimension do not view themselves as being in control of their health care. Feeling decidedly unhealthy, low scorers have relinquished control. With no interest in trying exercise or a healthful diet before turning to a prescription drug, low scorers willingly rely on such drugs to feel better. Low scorers do not equate taking such drugs with giving up control over their health.

Identifying those who score high or low on this dimension is critical in understanding the health motivations of those 40 and older. While empowering some-one to assume responsibility for his or her health is im-portant, it is also important to stress a balance between taking care of one's health and choosing to be one's own doctor.

RELATIONSHIPS

Demographics

A significant relationship exists between five demographic measures and this dimension: age, in-come, years of education, and gender or the number of children in the household.

Our research shows that the younger the person within the population of those 40 and older in the U.S., as well as the greater the income or years of education, the higher the score on the Self-determination dimen-sion. In addition, higher scores on the Self-determination dimension correlate with fewer children living in the household.

Men have higher scores on this dimension than women. This finding is not surprising. Other research has shown men less likely to visit a doctor than women, thus retaining control of their health.

Good health habits

The higher the score on the Self-determination di-mension the lower one's body mass index (BMI) or the more frequently one exercises at an aerobic level each week.

There is no difference between the scores of smok-ers and non-smokers on the Self-determination dimen-sion.

SELF-DETERMINATION FREQUENCY OF AEROBIC EXERCISE WEEKLY

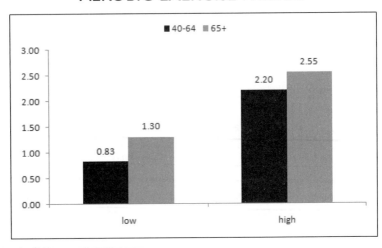

Figure 9-1: Persons with high scores on this dimension exercise more times per week at an aerobic level as compared to those with low scores.

Use of health-related services, products

The lower a person's score on the Self-determination dimension, the more a person has made use of medical services and products. These services and products include both daily use of OTC and prescription drugs, as well as the number of in- and outpatient hospital days over the past two years, and the number of doctor visits annually. In contrast, the reverse of all of these positions is true for those with higher scores on this dimension.

SELF-DETERMINATION
AVERAGE NUMBER OF RX TAKEN DAILY

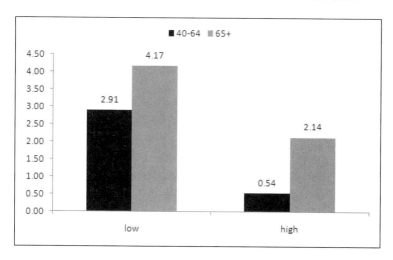

Figure 9-2: *Those with low scores on this dimension take a far greater number of prescription drugs daily as compared to those with high scores. Those 40-to-64 with low scores on the Self-determination dimension take a greater number of prescription drugs as compared to those who are 65+ and have high scores.*

Impact of disease on scores

Among the 16 chronic diseases we track, those with *none* of these diseases have higher scores on this dimension as compared to persons who have anyone of these diseases. This finding echoes one mentioned below.

We have already noted that those with higher scores on the Self-determination dimension are younger. They have either not yet developed or have not yet been diagnosed with chronic, debilitating diseases.

In sharp contrast, those with a higher number of the

87

chronic diseases we track have lower scores on the Self-determination dimension. Whether they have allergies, angina, artery disease, arthritis, cancer, heart disease, glaucoma, depression, diabetes, high blood pressure, back problems, chronic migraines, sinus problems, stroke, or osteoporosis, those in this group believe factors outside of themselves determine their health.

Multiple chronic diseases

One analysis we conducted focused on a group of six chronic diseases, including cancer, depression, diabetes, and stroke. We found that when the actual number of these chronic diseases our respondents have is measured against their scores on the Self-determination dimension, scores on this dimension correlate with the number of diseases reported. That is, those with higher scores on this dimension report fewer chronic diseases from this group, while those with lower scores have greater numbers of these diseases.

Influencers on improving diet

Those who have reduced the food components of sodium, fat, sugar, cholesterol, and calories *on their own* have higher scores on the Self-determination dimension.

On the other hand, those who have reduced sodium, fat, sugar, cholesterol, caffeine, and calories *on a doctor's advice* have lower scores on this dimension.

Health insurance

Those who obtain health-care coverage from a managed care organization have higher scores on the Self-determination dimension in contrast to those not insured using this source.

In contrast, persons who receive health-care insur-

SELF-DETERMINATION
AVERAGE NUMBER OF CHRONIC DISEASES

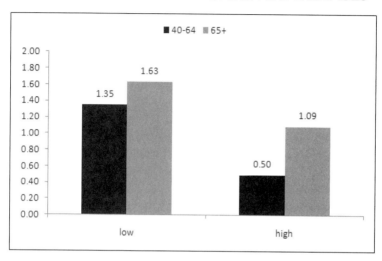

Figure 9-3: *Persons with low scores on this dimension have a far greater number of chronic diseases as compared to those with high scores. Those 40-to-64 with low scores on the Self-determination dimension have a greater number of chronic diseases as compared to those 65+ with high scores.*

ance from either Medicare or Medicaid have lower scores on this dimension.

Sources of information

Individuals who have used health magazines, books, or their spouse (among those who are married) for health information within the past 12 months have higher scores on the Self-determination dimension.

In contrast, persons who have used the following sources of health information within the past 12 months have lower scores on the Self-determination dimension: advertisements, whether on television, radio, or in magazines; health organizations; a doctor; a

89

nurse; pharmacist; an employer (among those who are employed); government publications; product information; an 800 number for information on a prescription drug; videotapes; or seminars on health topics.

Preventive health examinations

Those who have not had a Pap test (limited to females), a bone scan, cholesterol test, hemoglobin A1c test, or a blood pressure examination within the past three years have higher scores on the Self-determination dimension compared to those who have had these tests and examinations.

OTC drugs

Persons taking no OTC drugs on a regular basis or those who take energy boosters, hair growth remedies, herbal medications, or memory enhancers have higher Self-determination dimension scores.

In contrast, those who regularly take or use antacids, antihistamines, cold medications, cough syrup, headache remedies, laxatives, sleeping pills, pain killers, skin lotion for dry skin, or skin ointment for pain have lower scores on this dimension.

IMPORTANCE OF THIS DIMENSION

Scores on our Self-determination dimension show to what degree an individual believes he or she retains control over his or her health care. Is one's health controlled by internal or external factors? Who or what is responsible for one's state of health? Someone with a high degree of internal control will score high on our Self-determination dimension. These high scorers believe their own actions determine their state of health. Conversely, low scorers on our Self-determination dimension are convinced factors outside of themselves, whether a doctor, fate, or chance, are responsible for their health.

Studied for decades

The concept of the level of control one feels over one's health—or health locus of control—has been studied for over 40 years. "In recent decades, a great deal of research has linked internal locus of control to positive health beliefs and behaviors. While not all attempts to correlate the two have been successful, it is widely accepted that health-related locus of control is significantly associated with a variety of health behaviors and outcomes."[1]

Linked to health behaviors

For example, internal locus of control has been associated with the ability to stop smoking or to lose weight. A study of almost 12,000 persons in the United Kingdom showed that a group of lifestyle indicators, such as exercising and not smoking, were "positively associated with internal health locus of control scores, and negatively associated with scores on the chance and powerful others dimensions."[2] In another study on weight loss, those completing a behavior modification weight-reduction program with an internal locus of control had significantly higher weight loss than those with an external locus of control.[3]

Internal locus of control has also been linked to following a medical regimen. In studying patients recovering from an acute myocardial infarction (AMI) from the perspective of their locus of control, researchers found that based on "three highly intercorrelated physiological measures . . . externals were found to have worse prognoses than internals."[4] Another study, this one on dialysis patients, found that those patients

91

with an internal locus of control orientation showed "a higher rate of compliance to medication and dietary restrictions than those patients with an external locus of control."[5]

Who's in charge?

Our Self-determination dimension is important because it yields insights into a person's attitudes toward who or what is responsible for his or her health. Educational health messages can be developed based on these insights. It has been shown that targeted health messages have had better results in motivating behavioral changes than those directed to a general audience.[6] It has also been demonstrated that locus of control affects receptivity to tailored health education materials.[7]

The prevention of chronic disease, the preservation of good health, and the stabilization or improvement of chronic conditions all rest on the ability to craft targeted health education messages based on the individual's own motivations. Knowing a person's score on the Self-determination dimension is critical in shaping messages that are most effective for that individual.

REFERENCES

[1] Amy Mackey. "Power, Pessimism & Prevention: The impact of locus of control on physical health." *units.muohio.edu*. Miami University. Web. 15 June 2010.

[2] Paul Norman, et al. "Health Locus of Control and Health Behaviour." *hpq.sagepub.com*. Journal of Health Psychology 3.2 (1998): 171-180. Web. 15 June 2010.

[3] Birgitta Adolfsson, et al. "Locus of Control and weight reduction." *pec-journal.com*. Patient Education and Counseling 56.1 (2005): 55-61. Web. 15 June 2010.

[4] R. Cromwell, et al. "Acute Myocardial Infarction." *work-health.org*. Work Health Organization. Web. 15 June 2010.

[5] W.J. Wenerowicz, et al. "Locus of Control and Degree of compliance in Hemodialysis Patients." *informaworld.com*. Renal Failure 2.5 & 6 (1978): 495-505. Web. 17 June 2010.

[6] Cheryl L. Holt, et al. "Does locus of control moderate the effects of tailored health education materials?" *oxfordjournals.org*. Health Education Research 15.4 (2000): 393-403. Web. 15 June, 2010.

[7] Holt, et al.

93

Chapter 10

SEEKS HEALTH-RELATED INFORMATION

DIMENSION DESCRIPTION

Persons who score high on the dimension of seeking health-related information go out of their way to absorb such information from a variety of sources. These sources can include their doctor, the popular media, as well as the government. What matters in this dimension is the high scorer's receptivity to and interest in such information.

Those scoring high on this dimension reveal that as they've grown older their health has become a greater concern to them. In seeking health information, high scorers wish to reduce their concerns or anxiety about their health.

Conversely, those who score low on this dimension do not seek out information on health-related topics, nor do they pay attention to it. Advancing years have not made low scorers more concerned about their health. Since those who score low on this dimension have little interest in health-related information, it would be difficult to get them to focus on these types of messages.

This dimension indicates a consumer's or patient's fundamental receptivity to health-related information. In disseminating such information, it will be far more difficult to gain the attention of a population of low scorers on this dimension than of high scorers.

RELATIONSHIPS

Demographics

Those with lower levels of education and income have higher scores on the Seeks Health-related Information dimension. That is, those who are less educated see themselves as highly committed to searching for health-related information. No doubt some of their efforts are focused on their ailments.

In addition, the higher the score on this dimension, the older the individual. Women and persons who are single also have higher scores on this dimension. One profile of those with higher scores on Seeks Health-related Information is that of older females with lower incomes.

In contrast, men, those who are married, those who are younger, as well as those with greater numbers of children in the household have lower scores on the Seeks Health-related Information dimension.

Good health habits

The lower the score on Seeks Health-related Information the more frequently one exercises at an aerobic level each week. It may be that these frequent and intense exercisers do not believe they need more health-related information. They are already putting such insights to active use. It is possible they may also feel they are in good health.

In addition, smokers have lower scores on the Seeks Health-related Information dimension as compared to non-smokers. In this instance, it may be that cigarette smokers have a fatalistic view of their health, don't see a need for health-related information, or aren't concerned about the effects of smoking.

A higher score on this dimension is also tied to increasingly elevated BMIs.

Overall, our data shows that the higher score on this dimension the fewer of the three good health habits practiced.

SEEKS HEALTH-RELATED INFORMATION
PERCENT CURRENT SMOKERS

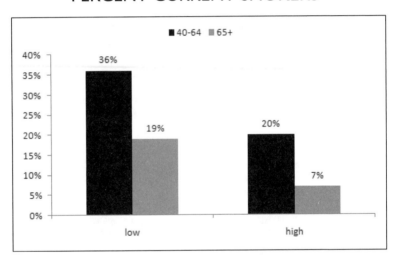

Figure 10-1: A greater percentage of those 40-to-64 are smokers as compared to those 65+. However, for both age groups, those with high scores on this dimension have a lower percentage of smokers .

Use of health-care services, products

Higher scores on this dimension are seen in five

areas of health-care utilization. The higher a person scores on this dimension the greater the number of prescription and OTC drugs taken on a daily basis, as well as the greater the number of in- and outpatient hospital days over the past two years, or the number of doctor visits per year.

Impact of disease on scores

Persons who report having allergies, angina, arthritis, congestive heart failure, depression, glaucoma, high blood pressure, osteoporosis, chronic migraines, sinus problems, or stroke have higher scores on the Seeks Health-related Information dimension.

SEEKS HEALTH-RELATED INFORMATION AVERAGE NUMBER OF RX TAKEN DAILY

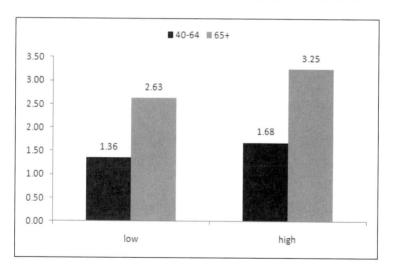

Figure 10-2: Those 65+ take a greater number of prescription drugs daily as compared to those 40-to-64. However, those with high scores for both age groups take a greater number of prescription drugs as compared to those with low scores.

97

Multiple chronic diseases

We examined the total number of chronic diseases our respondents have from a group of six. By comparing the number of these diseases to our respondents' scores on the Seeks Health-related Information dimension, we found the higher the score on this dimension the greater the number of diseases reported. Specifically, those with higher scores on the Seeks Health-related Information dimension report multiple chronic diseases.

Influencers on improving diet

Persons who reduced their intake of sodium, fat,

SEEKS HEALTH-RELATED INFORMATION
AVERAGE NUMBER OF CHRONIC DISEASES

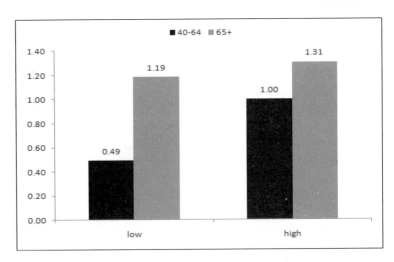

Figure 10-3: While a marginal difference exists between high and low scores on the Seeks Health-related Information dimension among those 65+, a dramatic difference is evident between low and high scorers in the 40-to-64 age group.

sugar, caffeine, cholesterol, or calories, whether *on a doctor's advice* or *on their own,* have higher scores on the Seeks Health-related Information dimension in contrast to those who did not do so.

Health insurance

Medicare enrollees, as well as those who have no health insurance, have higher scores on the Seeks Health-related Information dimension in contrast to those who obtain health insurance from other sources. We find persons covered by a major medical policy have lower scores on this dimension when compared to those who do not have such coverage.

Sources of information

Persons who have made use of information sources from the following list within the past 12 months have higher scores on the Seeks Health-related Information dimension.

These sources include health magazines; non-health-related magazines; newspapers; paid health newsletters; free health newsletters; advertisements on television, radio, and in a magazine; televised health programs; health organizations; books; a doctor; a nurse; relatives and friends; government publications; a pharmacist; an 800 number for information on a prescription drug; videotapes on health-care topics; health seminars; or product information.

Preventive health examinations

Both men and women who have had a bone scan or a hemoglobin A1c test within the past three years have higher scores on the Seeks Health-related Information dimension as compared to those who have not had these tests. In addition, women who have had a mam-

99

mogram within that time frame also have higher scores on this dimension.

OTC drugs

Persons regularly using acid blockers, antacids, antihistamines, cold medications, cough syrup, foot-care products, headache remedies, herbal medicines, laxatives, memory enhancers, pain killers, sleeping pills, skin lotions for dry skin, skin ointments for pain, or vitamin tablets or pills have higher scores on the Seeks Health-related Information dimension as compared to those who do not use such products.

Those who take either no OTC drugs or take potency enhancers have lower scores on this dimension.

IMPORTANCE OF THIS DIMENSION

The dimension of Seeks Health-related Information describes the act of collecting information related to health. This dimension does not encompass whether or not the material is actually understood. The issue of understanding health information is dealt with in a separate dimension also described in this book.

Need for information

Over the past decade, the great numbers of uninsured, the complexity of today's medicine, and the encouragement of employers and insurance companies are among the forces that have spurred the increase in individuals seeking health-related information. Considering the fact that Americans make an average of 3.8 doctor visits a year and that such visits last for an average of 22 minutes, the 84 minutes spent annually with a doctor seem inadequate to convey sufficient information and direction regarding the health problems or issues someone may have.[1, 2, 3]

It is true that Americans continue to rely on traditional sources of health information. For example, a Center for Studying Health System Change (HSC) study reports that health professionals, such as a doctor, are still the most frequently used source for health-related information with 86 percent of adults reporting using them. This study, however, also points out that increasing numbers of American adults rely on sources other than their doctor for health information. In 2001, 38 percent used a source other than their doctor for such information; by 2007 the percentage had climbed to 56 percent.[4]

Searches increase

It is also evident we are using the Internet in ever expanding numbers to gather information on health. For example, according to the Pew Internet and American Life Project, in 2000 just 25 percent of Americans looked online for health-related information. In 2009 it found that 61 percent of adults did so.[5] HSC found parallel results. Its studies show that the percentage of Americans using the Internet as a source of health information was 16 percent in 2001; by 2007 that percentage had doubled to 32 percent.[6]

Access differs

But seeking health information, and specifically using the Internet as a source for such information, is often hampered by a lack of access. Those with chronic disease "are significantly less likely than healthy adults to have access to the Internet (62% vs. 81%)." This lack of access curtails the use of the Internet for health information. While 66 percent of American adults with no chronic conditions have used the Internet as a source of health information, just 51 percent of those living with a chronic disease had done so. When adults living with two or more conditions are considered, the percentage is even lower (44 percent).[7]

In addition, the ability to use the Internet to retrieve health information is dependent on Internet savvy, something found far more typically among younger adults than those who are older. For example, the heaviest users of the Internet when seeking information about exercise and fitness are young adults. Although 57 percent of those 30 to 49 years of age have looked online for such information, 25 percent of those 65 plus have done so.[8]

Some left behind

As portions of the population increase their use of the Internet for health information, others are in danger of being left behind. The HSC study points out that "at least 50 million Americans who sought health information for themselves or others . . . did not conduct any health searches online."[9] For whatever reason, one sixth of the U.S. population has not conducted such searches. By not doing so, it is increasingly possible that this large portion of our population will remain uninformed of the latest health developments.

Besides the Internet searches done by the person for him- or herself, the previously mentioned Pew study also found that half of online health searches (52 percent) were done for someone else.[10] Regardless of the person for whom the searches are conducted, does the act of collecting health-related information in and of itself benefit someone's health? Does the very act of collecting such information influence health-related decisions or actions?

Positive results

In the Pew study, the majority (60 percent) of those

conducting Internet searches reported that such an impact does occur and that experiences are far more positive than negative. When asked about the impact of their last Internet search on a health-related topic, 13 percent reported a major impact, while 44 percent reported a minor impact. Another 41 percent reported no impact. The Pew study found that of the 57 percent of respondents reporting either a major or minor impact, 60 percent said that "information found online affected a decision about how to treat an illness or condition," while 38 percent said "it affected a decision about whether to see a doctor."[11]

In addressing the increase in the numbers of Americans seeking health information from any source, the HSC study found that a wide variety of Americans seek such information and that they "report positive effects from that information—effects such as increased understanding of conditions and treatments and a changed approach toward maintaining their own health."[12]

Subjective assessments

While these sources and others report the positive effects of such health information, one must remember that these are "subjective, self-reported assessments" that "may not represent actual improvements in consumer health behaviors or knowledge."[13] Considering also the immense amount of unreliable information on the Internet and in other sources, it may also be that health information seekers are not "taking a sufficiently critical approach to the information they come across."[14] Health information seekers may feel "empowered by the health information they find"; however, "some may be misled by less valid or credible sources."[15]

Quality concerns

In a study using the massive Health Information National Trends Survey data, 47.5 percent of the re-

103

spondents "strongly or somewhat agreed with the statement that they were concerned about information quality during their last search for cancer information."[16] Bradford W. Hesse, Chief of the National Cancer Institute's Health Communications and Informatics Research Branch of the Behavioral Research Program sees "a glut of information of uneven quality and readability, leading to 'caveat clicktor.'" He believes "Confusion is actually rising."[17]

Searches not easy

As large percentages of U.S. adults sought to find health information from whatever source, many found their searches to be a daunting experience. For example, among those searching for information about cancer more than a third (37.3 percent) reported that "their last search for cancer information took a lot of effort." In addition, more than a quarter of them (26.7 percent) agreed they "felt frustrated during their last search for cancer information."[18]

Impetus diverges

While some U.S. mature persons are charging ahead in their search for health-related information, the precise reasons for their quest can differ radically. Some may be seeking information for an acute condition, while others are interested in prevention, and still others want information on how to deal with a chronic disease they have already developed.

Beyond these root causes, our studies reveal a range of motivations that propel persons to seek or disregard health-related information. By understanding these motivations, health-related communications can be created using targeted messages and formats. In doing so, the appeal, as well as the effectiveness, of these health-related communications will be increased.

References

[1] Lena M. Chen, et al. "Primary Care Visit Duration and Quality." *archinte.ama-assn.org*. Archives of Internal Medicine 169.20 (2009): 1866-1872. Web. 7 July 2010.

[2] "Ambulatory Care Use and Physician Visits, Tables 1 & 2, Ambulatory Medical Care Utilization Estimates for 2006." Centers for Disease Control and Prevention. *www.nchs*. Web. 7 July 2010.

[3] Estella M. Geraghty, et al. "Primary Care Visit Length, Quality, and Satisfaction for Standardized Patients with Depression." *ncbi.nlm.nih.gov*. Journal of General Internal Medicine 22.12 (2007): 1641-1647. Web. 7 July 2010.

[4] Ha T. Tu and Genna R. Cohen. "Striking Jump in Consumers Seeking Health Information." *hschange.com*. Center for Studying Health System Change (HSC), Aug. 2008. Web. 3 July 2010.

[5] "The Social Life of Health Information." *pewinternt.org*. Pew Research Center, Internet & American Life Project, 11 June 2009. Web. 7 July 2010.

[6] Tu and Cohen.

[7] "Chronic Disease and the Internet." *pewinternet.org*. Pew Research Center, Internet & American Life Project, 24 May 2010. Web. 7 July 2010.

[8] "The Social Life of Health Information."

[9] Tu and Cohen.

[10] "The Social Life of Health Information."

[11] "The Social Life of Health Information."

[12] Tu and Cohen.

[13] Tu and Cohen.

[14] Tu and Cohen.

[15] Tu and Cohen.

[16] Neeraj K. Arora, et al. "Frustrated and Confused: The American Public Rates its Cancer-Related Information-Seeking Experiences." *ncbi.nlm.nih.gov*. Journal of General Internal Medicine 23.3 (2007): 223-228. Web. 7 July 2010.

[17] Peggy Eastman. "Study: Cancer Patients Increasingly Confused by Internet Health Information; Trust in Physicians Growing." *lww.com*. Oncology Times 7.7 (2010): 43-44. Web. 7 July 2010.

[18] Arora, et al.

Chapter 11

ABLE TO UNDERSTAND HEALTH INFORMATION

DIMENSION DESCRIPTION

Those with a high score on this dimension feel they can grasp and absorb health-related insights from various sources. They trust their sources of health information and believe their health issues and concerns are being heard.

High scorers believe they have the information they need to improve their health and act to do so. They are convinced that taking such actions will be beneficial. High scorers don't have to see or feel symptoms of a disease or condition before accepting a diagnosis.

In contrast, those scoring low on this dimension have difficulty grasping, understanding, and trusting health information. Whether or not they have reading difficulties, low scorers on this dimension exhibit attitudes impeding comprehension.

For example, their difficulty in understanding health information is enmeshed in a deep-rooted fatalism. Low scorers believe they will get a disease, such as cancer, regardless of their actions. In addition, low scorers believe they have a health problem only when they can see or feel the symptoms for themselves.

Low scorers have concluded that those to whom they turn for health information, such as their doctors, aren't providing it. When they attempt to communicate their health concerns or symptoms to their physician, they feel rebuffed.

Providing information on health-related topics is only the first step in ensuring that someone takes the required action. It is critically important to determine whether a consumer or patient actually understands the information.

Because of education, intelligence, language, or some other factor, a person may have a problem grasping information on health.

Our motivational dimension adds an additional perspective. The ability to understand health-related information can also be greatly enhanced or severely limited by some of the receiver's fundamental motivations.

These motivations encompass the nature of the relationship with the person delivering the information. In addition, this dimension reveals that the receiver's motivations regarding the value of health-related information and his or her willingness to act on it can affect whether or not it is understood.

RELATIONSHIPS

Demographics

Within those 40 and older in the U.S. population, years of education, as well as income, correlate positively with scores on the Able to Understand Health Information dimension. The higher one's level of education and income, the higher the score on this dimension.

Age is negatively correlated. Compared to younger

people, older people believe they are less able to under-stand health information.

In addition, the number of children in the household is positively correlated with scores on Able to Under-stand Health Information. That is, as the number of children in the household increases, the greater one's belief that one can understand health-related informa-tion. We believe this relationship is a function of age.

Higher scores are also seen among those who are married as compared to single persons.

Good health habits

We studied three major determinants of a healthy lifestyle: a normal weight defined by body mass index (BMI), the number of times per week one exercises at

ABLE TO UNDERSTAND HEALTH INFORMATION YEARS OF EDUCATION

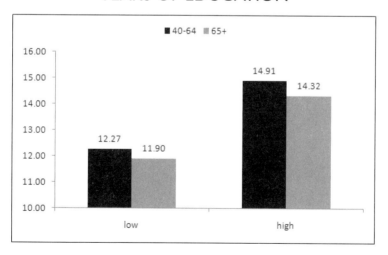

Figure 11-1: *Those with high scores on the Able to Under-stand Health Information dimension have more years of edu-cation as compared to those with low scores.*

109

an aerobic level, and not smoking.

Higher scores on Able to Understand Health Information are correlated with a higher BMI. It is troubling that those who believe they can comprehend health information are more likely to weigh more. It is clear that thinking one is able to understand health information, such as the need to maintain a normal body weight, does not translate into making the healthful decisions necessary to do so.

Higher scores on this dimension also correlate with the number of times one exercises per week at an aerobic level. The higher one's score on this dimension, the greater the number of times one exercises aerobically.

Higher scores on the Able to Understand Health

ABLE TO UNDERSTAND
HEALTH INFORMATION
PERCENT CURRENT SMOKERS

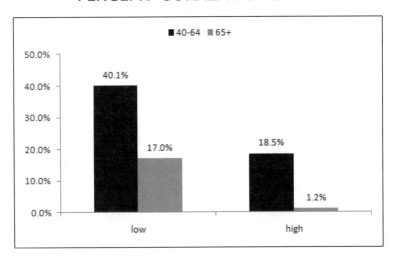

Figure 11-2: Within both age groups, those with low scores on this dimension have a higher percentage of smokers, as compared to those with high scores.

Information dimension among non-smokers suggest that communication campaigns on smoking cessation have been successful.

In contrast, the lower scores on this dimension among current smokers underscores the difficulty they will have in understanding smoking cessation messages. Smokers' belief that they have difficulty understanding health-related information could act as a roadblock to smoking cessation.

Scores on the Able to Understand Health Information dimension do not predict the number of the three good health habits an individual practices.

ABLE TO UNDERSTAND HEALTH INFORMATION FREQUENCY OF AEROBIC EXERCISE WEEKLY

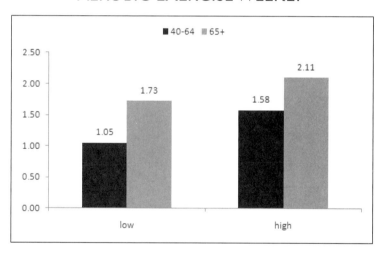

Figure 11-3: Persons 65+ exercise more times per week than those 40-to-64. However, those with high scores on this dimension exercise more frequently than those with low scores.

Use of health-care services, products

The Able to Understand Health Information score is negatively correlated with the number of inpatient days spent in a hospital over the last two years. That is, the higher one's score, the fewer days one has spent in a hospital over that time period.

In addition, higher scores on this dimension are also linked to fewer doctor visits per year. Those who believe they understand health-related information avoid both hospitalization as well as doctor visits, for whatever reason.

Impact of disease on scores

Persons with angina, artery disease, cancer, heart disease, as well as high blood pressure, are more likely to have lower scores on this dimension. We noted earlier the negative correlation between this dimension and age and education. Older components of the 40 and older age group are both more likely to have the severe conditions mentioned above and also believe they are less able to understand the information needed to deal with their illnesses.

On the other hand, persons with somewhat less severe maladies, such as allergies, osteoporosis, or back problems, have higher scores on Able to Understand Health Information.

Multiple chronic diseases

We examined a group of six chronic diseases, including cancer, diabetes, stroke, depression, and cardiovascular and upper respiratory conditions on the Able to Understand Health Information dimension.

We found that scores on this dimension correlate negatively with the number of diseases reported. That is, the higher the score on this dimension the lower the number of these chronic diseases.

Influencers on improving diet

Persons who have have reduced sodium, fat, cholesterol, or calories *on their own* have higher scores on this dimension as compared to those who have not made these changes on their own.

Those who have reduced the dietary factors of sodium, sugar, caffeine, or cholesterol *on a doctor's advice* have lower scores on this dimension as compared to those who have not acted on this prompting.

Health insurance

Persons receiving health insurance from managed care are more likely to have higher scores on this dimension compared to those persons who do not receive health-care insurance from this source.

We believe there are a few reasons for this situation, including the three which follow. In order to reach their objective of providing preventive care, managed care organizations stress patient education. It is possible that those who believe they are can comprehend health-related information migrate to managed care. Such organizations may also increase their members' abilities to comprehend health-related information through patient education efforts and disease management programs. And, finally, it may be that managed care organizations attract a younger and more educated population.

In contrast, a person receiving Medicare is likely to have lower scores on the Able to Understand Health Information dimension. We assume this finding is influenced by demographics. Medicare enrollees are preponderantly 65 and older, and, as we have shown, older people feel less able to understand health information.

113

Persons enrolled in a major medical policy have lower scores on this dimension as compared to persons not enrolled. In addition, those who have no health insurance also have lower scores on the Able to Understand Health Information dimension as compared to those who have health insurance from any source.

Sources of information

It should be no surprise that persons who believe they can understand health information are avid consumers of it and utilize multiple sources. Of the 21 sources of information we studied, wide-ranging consumers of 13 sources of health information have higher Able to Understand Health Information dimension scores as compared to those who do not use such sources.

Those persons who had read or viewed health information from health magazines; non-health-related magazines; newspapers; free health newsletters; advertisements on television, radio, and in magazines; health organizations; books; a doctor; the Internet (if they have access); relatives and friends; government publications; product information; as well as health seminars had higher scores on the Able to Understand Health Information dimension.

It is important to note that many of the sources of health information used by those with higher scorers on this dimension involve reading.

Preventive health examinations

Those who had a mammogram, Pap test (both limited to females), a cholesterol test, or a blood pressure examination within the past three years received higher scores on the Able to Understand Health Information dimension than those who had not had these tests.

OTC drugs

Those who take or use antihistamines, vitamin tablets or pills, or hair growth remedies daily have higher scores on this dimension as compared to those who do not take such drugs.

Those who use acid blockers, cold medications, cough syrup, foot-care products, diet pills, headache remedies, laxatives, potency enhancers, skin lotions for dry skin, or skin ointments for pain on a daily basis have lower scores on the Able to Understand Health Information dimension as compared to those who do not take or use these products.

IMPORTANCE OF THIS DIMENSION

Defining health literacy

The National Library of Medicine defines health literacy as "The degree to which individuals have the capacity to obtain, process, and understand basic health information and services needed to make appropriate health decisions." This definition was used by the Centers for Disease Control (CDC) in its *Healthy People 2010* document.[1]

The Institute of Medicine underscores the fact, however, that "there is more to health literacy than reading and understanding health information. Health literacy also encompasses . . . factors that influence the expectations and preferences of the individual . . . . Health care practitioners literally have to understand where their patients 'are coming from'—the beliefs, values, and cultural mores and traditions that influence how health care information is shared and received."[2] And it is these beliefs and values that are captured in our two motivationally based dimensions regarding health information.

Two dimensions

As we note in the Seeks Health-related Information chapter, our seven critical health dimensions include two separate dimensions covering health information. One of our dimensions focuses on the extent to which one feels he or she seeks health information. The second rests on the conviction that one can comprehend such information.

One can score high or low on either the Seeks Health-related Information or the Able to Understand Health Information dimensions. High scores on both of these dimensions represent the optimal situation. Although our two dimensions are distinct and not statistically related, when considered together they represent what is defined as health literacy.

Effects of low health literacy

The Committee on Health Literacy, Board on Neuroscience and Behavioral Health, at the Institute of Medicine of the National Academies cites studies showing that "Individuals with inadequate health literacy as currently measured report less knowledge about their medical conditions and treatment, worse health status, less understanding and use of preventive services, and a higher rate of hospitalization than those with marginal or adequate health literacy."[3] In terms of patient compliance and prevention, the Institute of Medicine finds that "Adults with limited health literacy, as measured by reading and numeracy skills, have less knowledge of disease management and of health-promoting behaviors . . . ."[4]

Those who have a low level of health literacy typically do not understand what their doctor is telling them, do not take medications properly, fail to show up for appointments, and do not understand their medical insurance policies. Those in this group test below high school level in their reading skills. An estimated 40 million U.S. adults "have difficulty finding information in unfamiliar or complex texts such as newspaper articles, editorials, medicine labels, forms, or charts."[5]

Because medical and health materials are typically written at far above the high school level, experts conclude that 90 million adults may lack the needed literacy skills to use the U.S. health system effectively.[6] An even bleaker picture is presented by the National Assessment of Adult Literacy which found that only "12 percent of adults have *Proficient* [italics theirs] health literacy . . ."[7] It could be that nearly nine out of ten adults lack the skills needed to manage their health and prevent disease.

Costs of low health literacy

At a time when the U.S. is threatened by increasing health-care costs, it is important to note that the "annual health care costs for individuals with low literacy skills are *4 times higher* than those with higher literacy skills."[8] And at a time when prevention is a central strategy in dealing with these rising health-care costs, those with limited health literacy skills are "associated with an increase in preventable hospital visits and admissions. . . . Persons with limited health literacy skills make greater use of services designed to *treat* complications of disease and less use of services designed to *prevent* complications."[9]

Affecting access

The lack of such literacy skills has several negative results with far-reaching consequences for one's health. Knowledge of what is covered by one's health-care plan, for example, is necessary in order to access services. But in a "survey of nearly 2,100 covered workers, Watson Wyatt found that a top challenge for 43

117

percent of workers is understanding what their health-care plan covers. Moreover, less than half are confident explaining common health benefit terms, such as co-pay or deductible, to a friend or coworker. And fewer than one in four feels comfortable describing health savings accounts, coinsurance and terms such as for-mulary and center of excellence."[10]

Benefits of high health literacy

In contrast to those with low levels of health liter-acy, persons functioning at a higher level have "shorter hospital stays, less complications, have less stress re-lated to the treatment, and feel more satisfied about their care," according to the Joint Commission on Health Care.[11] We see then that both the ability to stay healthy and to treat an illness once one is sick is heav-ily dependent on a high level of health literacy.

Improved basic literacy skills offer a substantial health benefit, as well as a cost savings, as illustrated by a study conducted at the UCLA/Johnson & Johnson Health Care Institute.

After participating in a Head Start health literacy program, families having a total of 20,000 children changed how they used health-care services. "Hospital emergency room[s] dropped by 58 percent and visits to a clinic dropped by 42 percent as parents learned to deal with their children's fevers, colds, and earaches at home." These changes in behavior stemming from im-proved health literacy added up to "a potential annual savings to the U.S. Medicaid program of about $5.2 million annually in direct costs . . ."[12]

It is apparent "Health literacy can save lives, save money, and improve the lives and well-being of mil-lions of Americans," as the former U.S. Surgeon Gen-eral Richard Carmona has noted.[13] Because of its tre-mendous potential impact, improving health literacy was one of the goals of *U.S. Healthy People 2010,* and it has been retained as one of the objectives for 2020.

The two motivationally based dimensions we have developed on health information underpin our effort to understand the motivational facets of health literacy. Scores on this dimension quickly and reliably reveal patients' perceptions of how well they believe they understand health information. In addition, this measurement indicates possible attitudinal barriers to comprehension, as well as discrepancies between perception and reality. Some patients may believe they understand health information, but actual assessments may reveal they do not.

REFERENCES

[1] Lynn Nielsen-Bohlman, et al eds. "Health Literacy: A prescription to end confusion." Washington, D.C.: The National Academies Press, 2004. Print.

[2] "What Did the Doctor Say?: Improving Health Literacy to Protect Patient Safety." *jointcommission.org.* The Joint Commission, 2 Feb. 2007. 12 Nov. 2010.

[3] "Health Literacy: A prescription to end confusion," 82.

[4] "Health Literacy: A prescription to end confusion," 83.

[5] "Health Literacy: A prescription to end confusion," 67.

[6] "Health Literacy: A prescription to end confusion," 67.

[7] "The Health Literacy of America's Adults: Results from the 2003 National Assessment of Adult Literacy." *nces.ed.gov.* National Center for Education Statistics, 2003. Web. 1 Dec. 2010.

[8] "Health Literacy: Statistics At-A-Glance." *npsf.org.* Partnership for Clear Health Communication, National Patient Safety Foundation, June 2008. Web. 10 July 2010.

[9] "Fact Sheet: Health Literacy Basics, Quick Guide to Health Literacy." U.S. Department of Health & Human Services. *health.gov.* Web. 10 July 2010.

[10] "Many Workers Struggle with Basic Health Benefit Terms, Watson Wyatt Survey Finds." *insurancenewsnet.com.* Insurance News Net, 9 July 2007. Web. 10 July 2010.

[11] Donna Theobald. "Medical Tips: How to be an informed patient." *essortment.com.* Web. 10 July 2010.

[12] "Health Care Information and Health Literacy." *jnj.com.* UCLA Johnson & Johnson Health Care Institute. Web. 10 July 2010.

[13] Richard H. Carmona. "Health Literacy in the Public Health Service." *dcp.psc.gov.* Web. 10 July 2010.

Chapter 12

CONCERNED OVER COST

DIMENSION DESCRIPTION

Those who score high on this dimension are exceedingly concerned about the cost of health care. For example, high scorers are committed to economizing on the cost of their drugs. With this in mind, those who score high on this dimension are convinced generic drugs are as good as branded ones, and they search out the least expensive options.

On the other hand, those who score low on this dimension have little concern over the cost of health care. They are not committed to saving money on prescription drugs and don't favor the use of generics or other low-cost options.

Besides the obvious need to find out how a patient will pay for his or her necessary health care, a high or low score on the Concerned over Cost dimension establishes the patient's perception of his or her ability or willingness to pay for medical care.

RELATIONSHIPS

Demographics

As one would expect, the Concerned over Cost dimension correlates negatively with income. As incomes rise, scores on Concerned over Cost dimension decrease. These scores also decrease as the number of children in the household diminishes. Other demographic variables such as age or marital status were not significantly related to this dimension.

Good health habits

A higher concern over health-care costs is found among those who smoke cigarettes as contrasted to

CONCERNED OVER COST
ANNUAL HOUSEHOLD INCOME

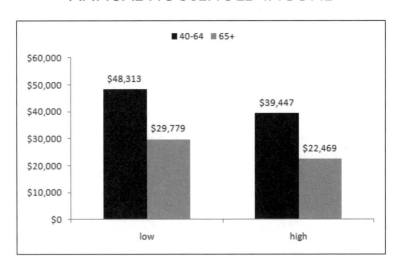

Figure 12-1: *Persons 40-to-64 have higher household income than those 65+. In addition, regardless of age, those with high scores on the Concerned over Cost dimension have lower incomes as compared to those with low scores.*

those who do not smoke. It could be smokers are already experiencing escalating health-care costs due to smoking-related illnesses. This conclusion is supported by a finding mentioned in the section found below on the impact of disease on scores.

Higher scores on the Concerned over Cost dimension are linked to higher measures of BMI, as well as a lower number of aerobic exercise sessions per week.

Use of health-care services, products

Scores on the Concerned over Cost dimension have no statistical relationship to the number of annual doctor visits, number of prescription or OTC drugs taken

CONCERNED OVER COST
PERCENT CURRENT SMOKERS

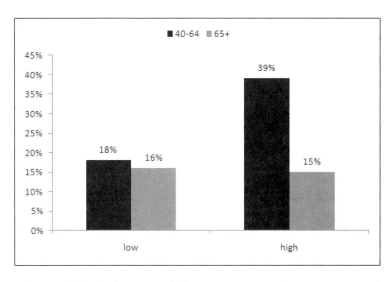

Figure 12-2: A dramatic difference exists in the percentage of smokers in the 40-to-64-age group on the Concerned over Cost dimension between those with high and low scores. There is no difference in the percentage of smokers in the 65+ age group between high and low scorers on this dimension.

123

daily, or inpatient days spent in a hospital over the past two years. Those with higher scores on this dimension are tied to increased numbers of outpatient hospital days.

Impact of disease on scores

Persons with diabetes, depression, or back problems have higher scores on the Concerned over Cost dimension. On the other hand, those with glaucoma or stroke have lower scores on this dimension as compared to those who do not have these diseases.

Multiple chronic diseases

In order to calculate each individual's number of chronic diseases, we focused on six. We grouped chronic diseases related to the heart into one category. The remaining five diseases included diabetes, depression, cancer, stroke, and upper respiratory conditions.

In examining the actual number of chronic diseases our respondents have against their scores on the Concerned over Cost dimension, we found that scores on this dimension correlate positively with the number of diseases reported. Specifically, those with higher scores on this dimension report multiple chronic diseases.

Influencers on improving diet

Persons who have reduced cholesterol and calories *on their own* have higher scores on the Concerned over Cost dimension as compared to those who have not reduced these food components. At the same time, those who reduced the dietary factors of fat and sugar *on a doctor's advice* have higher scores on this dimension compared to those who have not cut back on them.

Those who have reduced sodium due to *their doc-*

CONCERNED OVER COST
AVERAGE NUMBER OF CHRONIC DISEASES

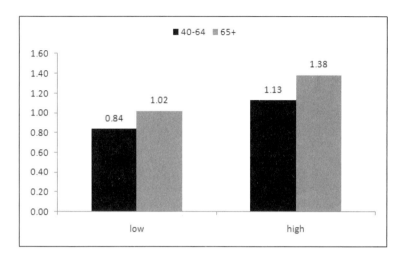

Figure 12-3: Those with high scores on this dimension report a higher number of chronic diseases as compared to those with low scores. Those with high scores among those 40-to-64 have a similar number of chronic diseases as compared to those 65+ with low scores.

tor's advice or caffeine *on their own* have lower scores on the Concerned over Cost dimension.

Health insurance

Those with health insurance coverage from Medicare or a major medical policy have lower scores on the Concerned over Cost dimension as compared to those not insured by such types of insurance.

In contrast, the uninsured have higher scores on the Concerned over Cost dimension in comparison to those who are insured.

Sources of information

Persons who relied upon non-health magazines, newspapers, or a nurse over the past 12 months as a source of health information have higher scores on the Concerned over Cost dimension as compared to those who did not use these sources. Most of these sources are both accessible and low in cost. Based on our insights, it would be reasonable, for example, for a government agency or health-insurance company to provide free health information through a sponsored newspaper column.

In contrast, those who have obtained health information from health magazines, the Internet (limited to those with access), and videotapes have lower scores on the Concerned over Cost dimension. We view these sources of health information as more specialized and costly than those listed above.

Preventive health examinations

Those who have had a Pap test (limited to females), a cholesterol test, a hemoglobin A1c test, or a blood pressure examination within the past three years have higher scores on the Concerned over Cost dimension as compared to those who have not had these tests or examinations.

OTC drugs

Persons who say they take no OTC drugs on a regular basis have higher scores on the Concerned over Cost dimension compared to those who rely on such medications.

Those who take acid blockers, antihistamines, laxatives, pain killers, skin ointments for pain or sleeping pills also have higher scores on this dimension.

Persons who regularly use diet pills are the only

OTC users with lower scores on this dimension.

IMPORTANCE OF THIS DIMENSION

In the U.S. a concern over the cost of health care is not limited to those without health insurance. "If you're sick enough long enough, you're in deep trouble in our society," said David Himmelstein, an associate professor of medicine at Harvard Medical School, and one of the authors of a study by Harvard University legal and medical researchers on how medical bills impact personal bankruptcy rates.[1] While our research shows the uninsured have the highest scores on our Concerned over Cost dimension, they are by no means the only ones with this concern.

Not enough insurance

In 2010, 52 million Americans under 65 were estimated to lack health insurance.[2] This group was joined by another "roughly 25 million Americans [who] are underinsured—in addition to paying a policy premium, they spend more than 10 percent of their income on out-of-pocket medical costs."[3] A 2008 study by the Commonwealth Fund added the uninsured to the underinsured and found that 42 percent of the U.S. under 65 population "had either no insurance or inadequate insurance in 2007, up from 35 percent in 2003."[4]

The results of a lack of health insurance, as well as inadequate health insurance, are seen in the fact that "In 2007, an American family filed for medical bankruptcy every 90 seconds. Three quarters of those families were insured, according to a Harvard study."[5] Beyond the uninsured and the underinsured, surveys have also found a great deal of concern over health-care costs among those who are currently insured through plans obtained at work.

Workers are worried

A 2007 survey by Watson Wyatt of 2,100 U.S. workers found that "More than one-third (35%) of respondents are concerned that a major medical expense would ruin them financially. . . . About one in four workers also reported higher stress levels due to rising health care costs."[6] The employees' concern over health-care costs springs from reality. For the past ten years, employees have seen increased cost sharing reflected in such things as higher co-payments, reduced subsidies for dependents, and tiered pharmaceutical benefits.

Cutting health care

Those who score high on our Concerned over Cost dimension may engage in a number of behaviors: avoiding doctor visits, putting off preventive or non-acute tests and procedures, not filling or refilling prescriptions, or cutting pills in half or taking fewer of them.

The Great Recession prompted an increase in behaviors explained by the Concerned over Cost dimension. Reacting to the cost of branded prescriptions, Wolters Kluwer Health reported that U.S. patients in the fourth quarter of 2008 "failed to fill 6.8 percent of brand-name prescriptions their doctors requested." This percentage represents a 22 percent increase over the first quarter of 2007.[7]

A study by Kurt Salmon Associates found that "Prescription drug users are increasingly price sensitive. In January 2009, 20 percent of prescription drug consumers cited price as a reason for switching retailers." This percentage represents an increase from 16 percent in 2008.[8]

In a 2008 study of 250,000 insured employees, knee replacements per 1,000 people fell 18.6 percent between March 2007 and March 2008, while Pap smears fell 6 percent.[9] The trend continued in the second quarter of 2010 when "Insurers, lab-testing companies, hospitals and doctor-billing concerns say that patient visits, drug prescriptions and procedures were down . . . from year-ago levels."[10]

Too late after too little

Deferring health care can lead to the late diagnosis of a disease or condition, as well as treatments that are unsuccessful because they are not fully applied. A diagnosis late in the stage of a disease or condition can lead to fewer treatment options, greater pain, increased disability, higher treatment costs, and death as a more certain and earlier outcome. "Health-policy experts say that . . . As more people forgo screenings or wait until minor medical problems blow up into serious complications, hospital and emergency-room admissions could eventually spike."[11]

For some, cost nonissue

On the other hand, those who score low on the Concerned over Cost dimension may find themselves taking medications unnecessarily. They may grow to rely on pills and procedures to restore their health, rather than preventing health problems in the first place. A lack of concern over the cost of procedures or examinations may make a patient or consumer more willing to have unnecessary tests and exams. Without giving much thought to the risks involved, patients may have unneeded tests that are themselves harmful or misleading.

The lack of concern over health-care costs is evident in a study conducted in 2005 in which only five percent of persons covered by an employer health-care plan had ever "used an online cost or quality comparison tool . . . ." and that "79 percent of the respondents [had] never learned the cost of a medical service or learned it only after they paid for it."[12]

Not aware of costs

This study found that consumers have little grasp of the true cost of medical services and products. Respondents who were able to give the correct cost of a new Honda Accord within five percent and the actual cost of a Bose Wave Music System within six percent, were not so successful with medical costs. They overestimated the cost of a visit to the emergency room by 70 percent and underestimated the cost of a four-day hospital stay by 61 percent. With such a weak grasp of the true cost of medical services, consumers may not be motivated to reduce health-care costs through activities that would preserve good health and prevent or control disease.

The Concerned over Cost dimension is of critical importance to the health of those 40 and older, whether they are insured, underinsured, or uninsured. The cost of health care can have a deleterious effect not only on one's health, but also on one's financial survival. This point is no doubt appreciated by those who score high on this dimension. Conversely, if the unnecessary use of health care is to decrease, then those who score low on this dimension will need to be educated about the true cost of the services and products they consume and the economic impact of their consumption.

REFERENCES

[1] Reed Abelson. "U.S. medical bills can cripple the insured." *nytimes.com*. New York Times, 3 Feb. 2005. Web. 5 March 2005.

[2] Todd P. Gilmer and Richard G. Kronick. "Hard Times and Health Insurance: How Many Americans Will be Uninsured by 2010." *healthaffairs.org*. Health Affairs 28.4 (2009): w573-w577. Web. 15 June 2010.

[3] James Oliphant and Kim Geiger. "Plenty of healthcare aches and pains." *latimes.com*. Los Angeles Times, 9 Sept. 2009. Web. 15 June 2010.

[4] Cathy Schoen, et al. "How Many are Underinsured? Trends Among U.S. Adults, 2003 and 2007." *healthaffairs.org*. Health Affairs 27.4 (2008): w298-w309. Web. 15 June 2010.

[5] Oliphant and Geiger.

[6] "Employee Perspectives on Health Care: Voice of the Consumer." *wyattwatson.com*. Wyatt Watson Worldwide, Jan. 2007. Web. 15 June 2010.

[7] Jonathan D. Rockoff. "Many Drug Prescriptions Are Now Going Unfilled." *online.wsj.com*. Wall Street Journal, 8 April 2009. Web. 15 June 2010.

[8] "Consumers Spending Less on Prescription Drugs." *pharmavoice.com*. PharmaVOICE, April 2009. Web. 15 June 2010.

[9] Vanessa Fuhrmans. "Consumers Cut Health Spending, As Economic Downturn Takes Toll." *online.wsj.com*. Wall Street Journal, 22 Sept. 2008. Web. 17 May 2010.

[10] Avery Johnson, Jonathan D. Rockoff, and Anna Wilde Mathews. "Americans Cut Back on Visits to Doctor." *online.wsj.com*. Wall Street Journal, 29 July 2010. Web. 16 Nov. 2010.

[11] Fuhrmans.

[12] "Consumer Attitudes Toward Health Care." *greatwesthealthcare.com*. Great-West Healthcare, Aug. 2006. Web. 15 June 2010.

PART 3

Chapter 13

SEGMENTATIONS

Evolution of the dimensions

We derived the seven dimensions forming the Morgan-Levy Health Cube from our three separate segmentations on the health motivations of the 40-and-older U.S. population. Each segmentation focuses on a different aspect of health. In addition, each segmentation has multiple segments within it.

Three separate motivational segmentations

Our studies on the health-related attitudes and motivations of those 40 and older began with our Health segmentation covering general aspects of health. Our Health Information segmentation focuses on attitudes related to using health-related information: sources relied on, importance given to this activity, and whether such information is perceived as beneficial.

Our third segmentation, Health Compliance, examines attitudes toward such elements of compliance as following a doctor's instructions and control over one's health-care decisions. In all, 203 attitude statements were originally used in the creation of these segmentations.

Make up of a segment

Based on how they responded to the issues we presented in our surveys, persons were divided mathematically into segments or groups. Persons with similar responses to our attitude statements were placed in a segment. Each segment is, therefore, made up of persons who assigned similar importance to the issues we presented. By examining each unique segment, one can understand how the motivations of groups of persons 40 and older differ on issues related to their health.

Our next step was to extract the critical dimensions from our three health-related segmentations. When we mathematically reduced the issues across all three of our health-related segmentations, we isolated the seven critical dimensions forming the Morgan-Levy Health Cube. We went through this process so that our insights would be more accessible, as well as easier to use.

Two different perspectives

It is important to keep in mind that the dimensions and segments represent different perspectives. In the case of our segments, individuals within the U.S. 40 and older population are divided into groups with unique motivations. Persons whose answers categorize them as Faithful Patients, for example, believe they know what to do to live a healthful life, but procrastinate in taking action. In contrast, Proactives are convinced they are focused on living a healthful lifestyle.

In the case of the dimensions, each individual, regardless of which segment he or she falls into, is assessed by the seven primary issues resulting from our research. Each person, therefore, has a score on each dimension. An individual may have a low score on the Healthy Lifestyle dimension, a high score on Self-determination, a middle or average score on Seeks

135

Health-related Information, and so forth. As we've pointed out previously, each dimension exists independently of the others.

The dimensions are the primary feature of the Morgan-Levy Health Cube, which facilitates classifying and understanding an individual's health-related motivations. Understanding these motivations is key to creating targeted communications promoting behavior change. By aggregating responses to the Morgan-Levy Health Cube from large populations, such as employees or insured individuals, one can study and learn from their dominant dimensions.

Dimensions combine within segments

While the seven dimensions in the Morgan-Levy Health Cube can be combined in many different ways, our research to date has isolated 14. Our individual segments represent these 14 combinations. An understanding of which dimensions are dominant within each segment, gives us a richer and deeper understanding of the health-related motivations of persons 40 and older in the U.S. population.

For example, while both Trusting Believers, a Health Compliance segment, and External Health Actives, a Health Information segment, have high scores on the Trust in Doctors dimension, of the two segments only External Health Actives have similarly high scores on Seeks Health-related Information. By understanding these patterns, we gain a comprehensive view of how combinations of these dimensions manifest themselves in the 40-and-older U.S. population.

Discovering relationships

Our original focus in creating our three segmentations on health was to quantify them within the current population. In contrast, our interest in the dimensions was to discover and describe relationships based on our accumulated data.

Aging a factor in health

In the following chapters, we have illustrated the fact that age itself is a major influence on attitudes about health. It is also apparent, however, that motivations differ among individuals and that these differences shape health-related choices. Mature individuals, whether burdened with chronic disease or not, do become more concerned about their health as they age. But how they deal with aging and their health varies significantly according to their motivations.

Because 65 is the age at which persons typically enroll in Medicare, the charts we have included in Parts Two and Three show how the sizes of our segments change between two groups, those 40-to-64 and those 65 and older.

Chapter 14

THE HEALTH SEGMENTS

PROACTIVES

Those in this segment are intensely committed to exercise, eating a balanced diet, and avoiding foods high in fat. Proactives are convinced that taking such actions will have a positive effect on their health. They are also unique in their interest in collecting information on how to stay in good health. Proactives trust their doctors and respect the health-care system. They are compliant patients concerned with taking a prescription drug as directed.

Working to stay healthy

While one Health segment believes it gets sufficient exercise and another eats a balanced diet, only Proactives see themselves as actively taking both these actions. They are also the only segment avoiding foods high in fats. Proactives are distinguished from other Health segments by their intense commitment to all three of these actions. It is not surprising, then, that Proactives are very optimistic about staying in good health. Those in this segment can't think of additional things to do to improve their health.

138

At the heart of all the Proactives' preventive strategies is a very strong belief that these actions will have a positive effect. Proactives, for example, don't believe they are fated to get cancer. Along with Faithful Patients, Proactives are committed to getting an annual physical.

Underlying these actions is the Proactives' desire to live as long as they can, even if they are in pain. They are the only Health segment holding this view.

Using information on health

Proactives also differ from the other Health segments in researching and collecting information on how to stay in good health. While they say they don't understand most of what they hear about cancer, they aren't confused about what to do to avoid getting a serious illness. Compared to the other segments, they are the only ones viewed by their friends as experts on health-care topics.

Trust in doctors

Proactives work with their doctors, whom they trust. Those in this segment are the least apt to seek a second opinion. They want to feel their doctor is concerned about their state of health, and they believe they have no trouble finding doctors who will listen to them. Proactives view their doctors as knowledgeable about such things as drug interactions.

Prescription drugs beneficial

Proactives are convinced that prescription medications will have a positive effect. Perhaps their increasing concern about OTC drugs has led those in this segment to rely more heavily on prescription medications. As compliant patients, Proactives are careful to take medications as directed.

139

HEALTH SEGMENTS
PERCENT BY AGE

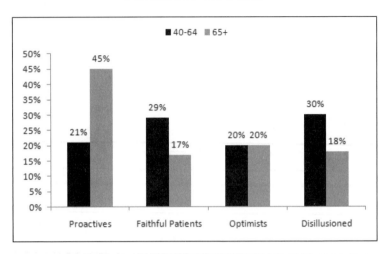

Figure 14-1: There is a significant shift in the proportions of Health segments between younger and older age groups. The percentage of Proactives increases in the 65+ bracket, whereas the numbers of Disillusioned and Faithful Patients decrease with age.

The medical system works

For Proactives, the medical system is functioning quite well. Proactives don't blame high medical costs on the system's inefficiencies or on lawyers pursuing medical malpractice cases. They believe there are government programs that would provide them with acceptable medical care. Proactives respect the system, denying they would experiment with drugs not approved by the Food and Drug Administration (FDA).

Committed to better hearing

While both Proactives and Faithful Patients, another

Health segment, are committed to having occasional hearing tests, the former are far more dedicated to taking care of their hearing. Of all the Health segments, only Proactives don't believe hearing aids make the wearer look old. They are also singular in thinking hearing aids are worth their cost.

Sufficient health insurance

Proactives are strongly convinced they have sufficient health insurance, regardless of the health problems they may face. They are the only Health segment with this view.

FAITHFUL PATIENTS

Those in this segment know what they should be doing to improve their health, but admit they don't take action. Since Faithful Patients don't take responsibility for their health, they are apt to turn to doctors, pharmacists, and medications to help them get better. They are the only segment that says it turns to religion in times of poor health. Faithful Patients are very interested in joining a health-maintenance organization (HMO) which would cover all of their health-care needs.

Not doing what they should

As they age, Faithful Patients have become increasingly concerned with their health. But this concern has not been translated into action. This segment admits they could do a great deal more to improve their health. Looking back, they wish they had eaten a more healthful diet when they were younger. Faithful Patients don't believe they eat a balanced diet, nor are they frequent dieters. They are very well aware of the fact they don't exercise enough to stay healthy. When they are sick, Faithful Patients turn to religion, the only Health seg-

141

ment to do so.

Perhaps the Faithful Patients' lack of follow-through regarding healthful behaviors is related to the fact that they have no desire to live a long life if they are in pain, something the Proactives willingly accept.

Trusting a medical approach

Since they don't take responsibility for their own health in very basic ways, Faithful Patients rely on doctors, pharmacists, prescription and OTC medications, and surgery to improve their health. Faithful Patients trust their doctors and consider it important to schedule an annual physical. Those in this segment rely on their pharmacist to keep them informed about OTC drugs. Faithful Patients advocate occasional hearing checks for older persons. If eye surgery would improve their vision, they would consider having it.

As do all the Health segments, Faithful Patients want their doctor to show concern about their state of health. While they trust their doctor, Faithful Patients would get a second opinion if faced with the need for a heart pacemaker. They prefer doctors who are specialists and feel very strongly that it is far better to have an eye examination from a medical doctor, or ophthalmologist, than from an optometrist.

Faithful Patients are careful to take a prescription medication as directed by their doctor. Taking these medications, they believe, is far better than having the disease. And Faithful Patients consider prescription medications to be effective and believe generic drugs work as well as branded ones.

Selecting health insurance

Faithful Patients are very interested in joining an HMO where all their health care needs would be met for one monthly premium. Although Faithful Patients are

142

somewhat concerned about having sufficient health insurance, they believe they are covered for any medical problem.

While blaming our litigious society and lawyers for high health-care costs, Faithful Patients would be the most prone of all the Health segments to sue a doctor if he or she made a mistake in treating them.

OPTIMISTS

Thanks to good luck, great genes, or infrequent health exams, those in this segment believe they are in terrific health. Optimists think that they rarely get sick. And if they were to get sick, those in this segment would think that there wasn't much they could have done to have avoided the illness. Optimists try to avoid taking prescription medications and see little need for health care delivered by an HMO: after all, they have no health problems.

Good genes, good luck

While they are committed to exercise, there isn't much more Optimists believe they can do to stay healthy. They aren't, for example, constantly dieting. Even with less than extensive efforts, Optimists are convinced they will remain in good health. Those in this segment reveal they rarely get sick. Even if they are sick, they might not know it: only those in this Health segment don't believe in having an annual physical. If they find out they have cancer, Optimists believe there was little they could have done to prevent it. Their fatalistic perspective appears to be related to a whole-hearted desire to live a full and happy life today and let tomorrow take care of itself. Looking back, they don't wish they had eaten a better diet when they were younger. Looking forward, they have no desire to extend their lives if it means living in pain.

143

Their avoidance in knowing about their health isn't related to feelings about doctors: Optimists trust doctors. They'd get a second opinion, however, before having a heart pacemaker implanted. Those in this segment prefer going to a medical doctor for an eye examination and would consider eye surgery if they were sure it would improve their sight.

Avoiding prescription drugs

Optimists shun prescription drugs, taking them only when it is critical, and avoid experimenting with OTC drugs.

Health-care perspectives

Since Optimists are in such good health, or at least believe they are, they have little need for health care delivered under the HMO concept. While guaranteed health care for everyone isn't something Optimists advocate, they don't see any government programs providing them with good health care. Like Faithful Patients, Optimists view a lawsuit-prone society as driving up health-care costs.

DISILLUSIONED

This segment's greatest concern is having insufficient health insurance. The Disillusioned are highly critical of today's health-care system and feel alienated from doctors. According to this segment, prescription medications are to be avoided if possible. One concern they have is that of harmful drug interactions. The Disillusioned would like to live a long life and act to improve their health. Their interest in achieving good health, however, is thwarted by their lack of access to health care.

Living a long life

The Disillusioned are concerned about living a long life and not just enjoying today. They believe certain actions, such as eating a balanced diet, will help them extend their lives and avoid diseases such as cancer. They seek information on how to stay in good health. Their desire for a long, healthy life is impeded, however, by their lack of access to health insurance. Of all the Health segments, the Disillusioned are most concerned about not having sufficient health insurance and worry about how they would cover a medical problem.

Health care in sorry state

Lacking health-insurance coverage, Disillusioned are sharply critical of today's health-care system, believing it is costly because it is inefficient. They think we need guaranteed health care for everyone. For those in this segment, HMOs are a welcome way of getting comprehensive health-care coverage.

Doctors are not to be trusted, say the Disillusioned, who have had difficulty in finding a doctor who will listen to them. Only they among the Health segments believe doctors don't know enough about how various medications interact. As do all of the Health segments, Disillusioned would like to find a doctor who is concerned about their health. While they too would seek a second opinion if their doctor recommended a heart pacemaker, they wouldn't sue a doctor who had made a mistake in treating them.

Avoiding medications

Disillusioned take prescription medications only when they have to and don't experiment with OTC drugs.

145

Chapter 15

THE HEALTH INFORMATION SEGMENTS

UNINVOLVED FATALISTS

Those in this segment have a fatalistic view of their ability to improve or preserve their health. They believe there is little they can do. Perhaps because of this viewpoint, Uninvolved Fatalists say they pay little attention to health information. They have a short-term perspective and have little concern for their future health. Although confused over health information and lacking confidence in making health-related decisions, Uninvolved Fatalists still view themselves as in charge of their health.

Fatalists to the core

As their name implies, Uninvolved Fatalists are fatalistic about their health. This pervasive fatalism affects every aspect of how they deal with their health, including whether or not they pay attention to health information. In their view, they will get sick no matter what they do. Uninvolved Fatalists believe there is nothing they can do to avoid diseases such as cancer.

146

Short-term perspective

Linked to the Uninvolved Fatalists' doomed view of their health is a short-term perspective. They focus on living life to the fullest now and not on the consequences of their actions. Making changes now so that they can be healthy in the years ahead is simply not a concern. They aren't thinking about living a long life.

Cost a factor

The cost of medical services also restrains Uninvolved Fatalists from getting the treatments and care they need. Whether because of a lack of commitment to better health or insufficient resources, only Uninvolved Fatalists do not believe it's important to have regular checkups from their doctor.

Vanity doesn't motivate

Unlike the other Health Information segments, Uninvolved Fatalists are not invested in their appearance. They aren't concerned about looking as young as possible and don't even care about looking good. Information about feeling and looking good is of no interest to those in this segment.

No interest in health information

With fatalistic and short-term perspectives about their health, Uninvolved Fatalists tell us they aren't interested in knowing about health or how to stay healthy. They are certainly not going out of their way to collect information about how to stay in good health. Even when being bombarded with health information, they don't pay attention to it.

The form or even source of health information won't change their lack of interest. Uninvolved Fatalists are oblivious to health information from the government. Health information on a television or radio show doesn't get their attention either. Even a popular television personality like Dr. Mehmet Oz could not cut through the Uninvolved Fatalists' lack of interest in health information. And health messages from the experts won't motivate them to change any destructive behaviors. Uninvolved Fatalists know their friends don't see them as knowledgeable about health care.

If they do read something about health and disease prevention, Uninvolved Fatalists are skeptical of it. It's only when they hear health information from many different sources that they may begin to believe it. And even

HEALTH INFORMATION SEGMENTS PERCENT BY AGE

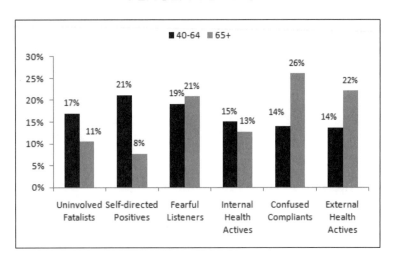

Figure 15-1: *At a statistically significant level, the proportion of the segments in each age group differs. Comparing the 40-to-64-year-olds to those 65+, Uninvolved Fatalists and Self-directed Positives decrease in size, while the sizes of the Confused Compliants and External Health Actives segments increase with age.*

148

then they are confused about what they should believe, particularly on what they should do to avoid a major disease.

Uninformed and confused, Uninvolved Fatalists see themselves as tentative in making choices about their health. When faced with making an important health decision, Uninvolved Fatalists are least apt to think through their alternatives and decide on a solution that makes the most sense to them. Instead, those in this segment would go by gut instinct in making major health-care choices.

Avoiding changes

Uninvolved Fatalists procrastinate about doing things to improve their health. Even when they decide to do something about their health, they don't follow through. They feel they don't do anything to avoid getting sick or to improve their health. Too busy to spend extra time on their own health, they reveal they are very caught up with taking care of others. Their perception that they currently enjoy good health could also encourage Uninvolved Fatalists to do nothing to benefit their future health.

Fatalistic, confused, and with no long-term perspectives on their health, Uninvolved Fatalists won't bother trying a new health idea. While Uninvolved Fatalists avoid doing things, such as exercise, that might improve their health, they continue other activities, such as eating high-fat foods, that they know might damage their health. Even reducing the stress in their lives isn't something they are willing to do.

Only a very strong argument would make an Uninvolved Fatalist even consider making health-related changes. Perhaps some unfortunate experience would serve as a wake-up call because Uninvolved Fatalists say they will only change after life teaches them a hard and nasty lesson. Yet this scenario seems doubtful: after an illness Uninvolved Fatalists tell us they try to forget everything about it.

149

Running the show

Another impediment to the Uninvolved Fatalists improving their health is their belief that they are in charge of their own health care. At the same time, those in this segment don't think they will know what to do to take care of their health-care problems. Uninvolved Fatalists admit that they are non-compliant and don't follow their doctor's instructions. While they take a passive position and don't argue with their doctor, they don't consider that he or she is always right.

For Uninvolved Fatalists, the best person to provide guidance regarding their health is themselves. When a doctor tells them they must quit smoking, a nurse advises them to loose weight, or they get any other advice that suggests they change what they are doing, they resent it.

SELF-DIRECTED POSITIVES

Those in this segment believe they are very smart people blessed with exceptionally good health. Because they have only a few vices, Self-directed Positives anticipate enjoying good health in the years ahead. Perhaps because of an optimistic view of their health, Self-directed Positives have little interest in health information. Those in this segment believe they are in charge of their own health care. Although they don't seek out health-care information, Self-directed Positives are supremely confident they will know what to do when faced with a health-care decision.

They are in charge

Self-directed Positives believe very strongly that they are the best persons to decide how to live a healthy life. Their health, they feel, is in their hands. They don't seek the counsel of friends and family before making a health-related decision. Resentment wells up in Self-directed Positives when someone tells them what they should do to take care of their health.

Convinced that they are very bright, Self-directed Positives see themselves as being able to handle any health-related problem. Besides this inner confidence, Self-directed Positives are also convinced they have the financial resources to handle any health situation.

When they have to make a decision regarding their health, Self-directed Positives believe they act in a very confident manner. After a decision has been made, those in this segment don't procrastinate, but instead follow through. Part of their motivation in doing so is that Self-directed Positives feel they don't have the time to get sick.

Luckily for them, those in this segment think they never get sick and view their bodies as being in very good shape. They are, in fact, so healthy they doubt that they will ever get cancer. The good health Self-directed Positives enjoy now, will, they think, last for a long time. After all, they tell us, they have only a few vices. But even if their lives are cut short, Self-directed Positives really aren't worried about the possibility of a shortened life span. They are fixated on living for the moment.

Not interested in health information

Since they believe they are currently in such good health, it isn't surprising that Self-directed Positives ignore health information, whatever its source or format. A thread of skepticism about health information also winds through the attitudes of Self-directed Positives. But whether presented in the mass media or a government pamphlet, Self-directed Positives stress they don't pay attention to health-related insights. Even if health information is presented on a favorite radio or television show, Self-directed Positives don't register interest in it. This lack of

151

interest isn't related to a feeling of confusion regarding health information. Self-directed Positives say they understand what they hear about cancer and don't feel confused about how to avoid major diseases.

FEARFUL LISTENERS

Fearful Listeners constantly absorb health-related information from a wide variety of sources. They may be motivated to do this because they are pessimistic about their current state of health and believe they are frequently sick. Fearful Listeners want to live a long life, but doubt they will achieve this goal. They see themselves as procrastinators when it comes to making health-related changes. Feeling in charge of their own health care, Fearful Listeners waffle on complying exactly with their doctor's instructions, and they resent those who advise them to change their habits.

Health information sponges

Fearful Listeners want to know a great deal about health. They constantly take in health-related information they receive from many sources. Whether this health information is from friends and relatives or found in a book or government pamphlet, Fearful Listeners consider all of these sources acceptable. If health information appears on the news or on their favorite radio or television shows, Fearful Listeners pay close attention to it.

Poor health an obstacle

While Fearful Listeners want to live a long life, they aren't sure they will achieve this goal. They are certain their health will fail and they will suffer some serious illness in the future. They are especially terrified of getting cancer. Fearful Listeners are pessimistic about the current state of their health, and perhaps their almost frantic efforts

152

to gather health-related information stem from this. They don't consider their bodies to be in very good shape and think of themselves as being sick frequently.

Not making changes

Constantly amassing information about health and, at the same time, pessimistic about the possibility of long-term survival, Fearful Listeners admit that they do not always act to improve or maintain their health. Considering the fact that they believe their health is poor and that their bodies are breaking down, it's not surprising Fearful Listeners say they have little interest in knowing what they must do to *stay* in good health. Regardless of all the information on health they gather, Fearful Listeners tell us they aren't open to trying new health ideas.

Fearful Listeners admit they are procrastinators, putting off changes that could improve their health. Even when they decide to do something to better their health, Fearful Listeners confess they don't follow-through. If something could damage their health, perhaps eating a massive dish of Ben & Jerry's high-fat ice cream, those in this segment say they would do it anyway.

Fearful Listeners admit they don't do anything special to avoid getting sick, not even reducing stress. They aren't committed to regular medical check-ups. The health information they accumulate may prompt Fearful Listeners to avoid following their doctor's instructions exactly. Resentful of anyone telling them to change what they are doing, they believe they are in charge of their own health.

Lacking confidence

Although they feel they should direct their own health care, Fearful Listeners don't do so with confidence. All the mountains of health-related information Fearful Listeners collect doesn't turn them into secure health con-

153

sumers able to handle any problem that might develop.

INTERNAL HEALTH ACTIVES

Those in this segment want to live a long, healthy life. They are convinced that what they do now will help them to attain their goal. Internal Health Actives are willing to sacrifice present pleasures in order to preserve their health for a long time. Interested in health-related information from a variety of sources, they say they act on this information in their everyday lives. Those in this segment are confident about how they handle health-care choices and are not at all confused about making them.

Long-term perspective

Internal Health Actives approach health from a long-term perspective. Rather than living life fully at the present time, they want to live a long life. Those in this segment believe that if they pay attention to health information today, they will be healthy in their old age. In addition, Internal Health Actives are convinced that making changes in their lives now will result in an old age blessed with good health.

Self-directed

Internal Health Actives are convinced their long-term goal will be realized only if they themselves make it happen through everyday choices. Those in this segment believe strongly that they themselves are responsible for their own health; they aren't waiting for miracles. Internal Health Actives have a regular schedule of medical check-ups with their doctor. They aren't willing to sacrifice their own health for that of others. Internal Health Actives aren't fatalists about their health; they don't, for example, believe that getting cancer is inevitable.

154

Interested in health information

Having accepted responsibility for their health, Internal Health Actives listen closely to a wide variety of sources for information and direction. Rather than resent someone who tells them how they can feel better, they listen. Internal Health Actives don't mind when someone advises them to change what they are doing.

Information that helps the Internal Health Actives attain their goals of good health and a long life is of interest to them, whether presented on a news program on television or radio, in a booklet from the government, or revealed by a local leader. Those in this segment are not skeptical about information on health and disease prevention and tend to believe most of what they read without having to see it in a variety of sources.

Internal Health Actives want information about what actions they can take to achieve better health. More than the other segments, they focus on learning about what they must do to be healthy. They both ferret out a great deal of information about how to stay in good health and also put it to use.

Not confused

Not confused about the health information they hear and read, Internal Health Actives make health decisions in a very confident manner. They know what to believe, and they understand what they have to do to avoid major diseases. A testimonial to the Internal Health Actives' scope and depth of knowledge about health is that their friends view them as experts in this area.

Making changes

Internal Health Actives act, not procrastinate, on the health information they obtain. Life doesn't have to punish those in this segment in order for them to change a de-

155

structive behavior, nor are strong arguments needed to convince them that they must make a change to improve their health. The enthusiasm Internal Health Actives have for making changes is seen in their willingness to try new health ideas. Internal Health Actives aren't too busy to spend extra time on their health; they make time to improve their health. Conversely, Internal Health Actives say they would stop doing unhealthy things, even if they enjoy them. They have reduced stress in their lives. Not surprisingly, they consider their bodies to be in really great shape.

CONFUSED COMPLIANTS

Those in this segment are confused about what they should do to avoid major diseases. They don't seek out health-care information so they can become knowledgeable consumers. Instead, they rely on their doctor's insights and direction. Confused Compliants don't procrastinate when it comes to taking care of themselves. They believe such efforts will have a beneficial effect on their health. Confused Compliants would like to live a long life, but do not view their present health as that good.

Not self-directed

Compared to the other Health Information segments, Confused Compliants are least apt to see themselves as very smart. They don't believe they can handle any health problem they may face. Confused Compliants are confused about health care and what they should do to avoid major diseases, especially cancer. They feel their friends do not regard them as informed about health-care matters.

Given their insecurities, it is understandable that Confused Compliants are the least apt to accept the idea that they are primarily responsible for making health-care decisions. They strongly deny they are the best person to decide how they can live a healthy life. While admitting their confusion regarding health care, Confused Compliants do not actively seek out information on health and admit they are only mildly interested in becoming informed. Even if their favorite radio or television show presents health-related information, Confused Compliants ignore it. Whatever health information they are exposed to, those in this segment view it with a skeptical eye.

Since they refuse to accept personal responsibility for their health, to whom or to what do those in this segment turn? When they or their loved ones are in poor health, one option for Confused Compliants is to turn to religion. Confused Compliants also shift responsibility to their doctor. Those in this segment tell us they do exactly as their doctor instructs, although they feel that he or she isn't always right. But whatever doubts Confused Compliants have about their doctor, they don't confront him or her on them.

Although the Confused Compliants don't know what to believe about health care, they feel they don't make health-related changes based on instinct. Rather, facts from experts, such as their doctor, motivate this segment to change. And because they rely on expert opinion, not their own, Confused Compliants feel confident when taking action on health-care matters.

Dedicated to improving health

Confused Compliants believe they are making special efforts to avoid getting sick. Concerned about living a long life, they are willing to give up things they know aren't healthful in order to achieve this end. One motivation for doing so is their perception of themselves as being frequently sick. They don't believe their bodies are in good shape. Those in this segment are also motivated to take care of themselves because they have to be able to take care of their family.

Confused Compliants don't procrastinate when it comes

to matters about their health. When they decide to do something to improve their physical well-being, they think they do a good job following through on it. Those in this segment say they have regular medical checkups and have reduced their stress levels. Confused Compliants believe that such actions will have beneficial effects, and, therefore, they feel somewhat optimistic about their health.

EXTERNAL HEALTH ACTIVES

Those in this segment are motivated by external forces to absorb health-related information and take care of their health. A prime reason External Health Actives want to stay healthy is so they can take care of their families. Weighed down with this responsibility, they are concerned with living long, healthy lives. External Health Actives collect an arsenal of health information from a variety of media sources and also from authorities, such as their doctor. Confident health-care consumers, External Health Actives believe their actions will enable them to stay healthy. If these efforts fail and they fall ill, those in this segment turn to an external force: religion.

External motivation

External Health Actives are motivated by external forces to take care of themselves. Because they feel they have to take care of their family, External Health Actives say they make a special effort to stay in good health. Perhaps because of this concern, External Health Actives are worried about living a long life and will give up present pleasures to achieve it. They are willing to listen when someone tells them about actions they should take now in order to enjoy a healthy old age.

Another external force in the care External Health Actives take of themselves is religion, something they turn to

158

when they or their loved ones are ill. External Health Actives also take care of themselves to preserve their outward appearance: they desire to look young. They are receptive to information about looking good, something that's a goal of theirs.

Interested in health information

Because External Health Actives feel they have to stay healthy, they pay attention to health information. While External Health Actives are open to a variety of sources of information on health, authoritative ones are especially important. A book or government brochure will get their interest. In their view, health information from a local leader, perhaps a local physician or state epidemiologist, can be relied on.

External Health Actives also pay attention to health information presented on radio or television programs, whether it is on the news or on one of their own favorite shows. External Health Actives aren't confused by health information; they are confident they know what to believe.

While they seek to become informed health-care consumers, those in this segment also accept direction from others. They don't consider themselves to be the highest authority in terms of figuring out the best way to live a healthy life. Faced with a health-care problem, External Health Actives use information to make decisions and don't rely solely on their feelings or intuition. Those in this segment think through all their options and come up with the one that makes the most sense. The solutions they consider may come from information they themselves have gathered or instructions from their doctor.

Pathways to health

Neither strong arguments nor adversity are needed to convince External Health Actives to improve their

159

health. Once they know what they have to do, they take immediate action. They don't feel they are too busy to take extra time to preserve or improve their well-being. Besides having regular medical check-ups, External Health Actives say they have given up unhealthy behaviors, even if they enjoyed them.

While External Health Actives are optimistic about their health, they also acknowledge the possibility that they will get a disease. They believe, however, that the special efforts they have made, such as reducing stress in their lives, will bring positive results. For example, External Health Actives aren't fatalistic about getting cancer.

Chapter **16**

THE HEALTH COMPLIANCE SEGMENTS

TRUSTING BELIEVERS

Trusting Believers transfer responsibility for their health care to their doctor in whom they have total faith and who, they believe, cares about them as people. This profound faith comes with an enormous expectation: their doctor knows exactly how to cure them. For their part, Trusting Believers exhibit a resilient compliance.

Faith in the doctor

Trusting Believers have a total, complete and unwavering belief in their doctors and in the prescription drugs they give them. Their motto: "Doctor knows best." Those in this segment follow their doctor's instructions exactly. In essence, they have turned over the management of their health to their doctors. In their view, it's the best way to protect their health: they believe doctors are the best resources for efficacious treatments and prescription drugs.

Trusting Believers have concluded that following their

161

doctor's advice is a cost-effective strategy. Doctors already know what to do — why research the topic on your own or second guess the expert? If a doctor prescribes a drug, Trusting Believers conclude they must need it.

A personal relationship

The reliance Trusting Believers place on their doctor stems from their feeling their doctor is concerned about their welfare. Perceiving they have a personal relationship with their doctor leads Trusting Believers to pay a great deal of attention to what their doctor tells them about their health. Those in this segment consider their doctor's advice and consultation to be of great benefit in understanding their medical problems. They are careful to read the information their doctor gives them and want frequent feedback — if not reassurance — about their condition.

Expectations are high

The confidence that Trusting Believers have in their doctor, however, comes with an immense expectation: their doctor must determine precisely what is wrong with them and be able to map out a detailed treatment plan. The physician in which the Trusting Believer has the greatest confidence is apt to be a specialist, not a general practitioner. When faced with a medical problem, Trusting Believers are also open to getting a second opinion.

Unwaveringly compliant

Trusting Believers reveal themselves to be highly compliant in several ways. They don't second guess their doctor and would not stop taking a medication without their doctor's approval. According to those in this segment, it is not their decision to stop taking a prescription drug. Nor are those in this segment tempted to stop and start taking a prescription drug depending on whether

162

HEALTH COMPLIANCE SEGMENTS
PERCENT BY AGE

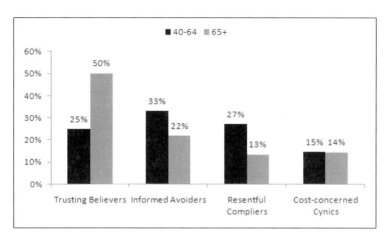

Figure 16-1: *There is a significant change in proportions between younger and older components of the Health Compliance segments. Trusting Believers 65+ increase with age,
while Informed Avoiders and Resentful Compliers decrease.*

or not they believe they need it. For them, adjusting the
dosage of a prescription is an unwise strategy. Even
when they don't see results, Trusting Believers would
continue taking a prescription drug.

Compliance results in good life

Trusting Believers are convinced that if they don't
follow their doctor's advice, they won't enjoy good
health. For Trusting Believers being compliant in taking a prescription drug will result in being healthy and
able to be with their family. Their high level of commitment to compliance in taking prescription drugs
also gives Trusting Believers a feeling they are doing
the most for their health. On a practical level, Trusting
Believers also want to get the most from their investment in a doctor's advice and prescriptions.

163

Reliance on prescription drugs

Taking a prescription drug for a health problem is the first line of defense for Trusting Believers. They wouldn't consider doing something else, such as taking a natural remedy or herb, before turning to a prescription drug. Having to take a prescription drug for the rest of their lives wouldn't deter Trusting Believers from starting the medication. Direct-to-consumer (DTC) advertising has a positive effect on Trusting Believers who feel more secure taking a prescription drug they have seen advertised on television. They do, however, view prescription generic drugs on par with branded ones.

Somewhat involved in care

Although reliant on their doctors to direct their care, Trusting Believers take some responsibility for their health by regularly checking their body for diseases. And they are the only Health Compliance segment that thinks it is a good idea to use a pill case marked with the days of the week to help them remember to take their medications each day.

INFORMED AVOIDERS

Informed Avoiders will do anything they can to avoid taking a prescription drug. They, not their doctors, are in charge of making final decisions regarding their health care. Informed Avoiders do everything they can to be informed about their health-care problems and conditions and use a variety of sources to achieve these ends. Of the Health Compliance segments, only Informed Avoiders believe they actually understand what their doctor tells them.

164

Avoiding prescription drugs

Informed Avoiders are the only Health Compliance segment committed to avoiding prescription drugs. They try other things before agreeing to take a drug. One way they avoid taking prescription drugs is through exercise and eating a healthful diet. Their avoidance of prescription drugs stems from worry over their long-term side effects, not their cost.

Informed Avoiders are concerned the cure offered by a prescription drug may be worse than the disease. Those in this segment feel very good about their lives, with the most positive views of all the Health Compliance segments. They are determined to do what they believe is most reasonable in order to preserve this feeling.

In charge of their health

In dramatic contrast to the Trusting Believers, Informed Avoiders believe they, not their doctors, direct their health care. Ultimately, Informed Avoiders want to make the final decisions regarding their health care.

Using health information

If Informed Avoiders have a health problem, they research it. They want to know every detail about their condition or disease, something they don't think takes too much time. Not only do they research their health problems, but, given a prescription, they check it out as well. Once they are comfortable they have the information to make an informed decision and thoroughly understand all the alternatives open to them, Informed Avoiders then formulate a plan to deal with a health problem.

165

A variety of sources

Informed Avoiders establish two-way communications with their health-care providers. On one hand, those in this segment don't have a problem being fully open and honest in their discussions with their doctors. At the same time, Informed Avoiders seek out and listen to a variety of experts, while still considering their health to be their own responsibility. If their doctor provides them with materials, they read them. They also pay close attention to what their doctor tells them about their health. Informed Avoiders find it helpful to get frequent feedback from their doctors.

For Informed Avoiders, the sources of health-related information may include several doctors: those in this segment are most committed to getting a second opinion about a health problem. And, like Trusting Believers, Informed Avoiders are more apt to rely on the advice of a specialist over that of a general practitioner. Informed Avoiders also see their pharmacist as a good source for information provided by the manufacturers of the prescription drugs they take.

It is extremely important to note that among the Health Compliance segments, only Informed Avoiders believe they understand what their doctor is telling them. This is not surprising: Informed Avoiders are the segment most committed to educating themselves on health issues. The implication, however, is that millions of patients in the other Health Compliance segments feel they don't understand what their doctors tell them, even though they may nod in agreement and ask a few questions.

Monitoring their health

Informed Avoiders pay a great deal of attention to how they feel. More than the other Health Compliance segments, those in this segment consider it important to check their bodies often.

RESENTFUL COMPLIERS

Resentful Compliers are stuck in a series of double binds. They distrust their doctors, but totally transfer responsibility for their care to them. While they don't believe what doctors tell them about their health conditions, they do little to become informed. Their non-compliant behavior is further fueled by their disbelief in having any disease whose symptoms are not seen or felt.

A failure to communicate

Resentful Compliers are trapped in a series of double binds. They have a profound distrust of their doctors, and, at the same time, they regard their doctor as the final decision maker regarding their health. Resentful Compliers also lack a strong commitment to seeking their own information on health issues. With few internal resources, Resentful Compliers say they would feel overwhelmed by a serious health problem.

Resentful Compliers are the only Health Compliance segment that believes doctors don't care about them as people, and they feel this very strongly. Only those in this segment believe doctors don't really listen to them.

Whether the cause or the effect, the profound lack of trust in doctors exhibited by Resentful Compliers shows up in deeply rooted communication problems. Those in this segment admit they don't understand when their doctor explains one of their medical problems.

While only slightly interested in researching their health issues, Resentful Compliers worry their own doctors don't understand their health problems as well as they do. And they do not see doctors as informed about the best medical practices.

Doctors, Resentful Compliers believe, are not to be trusted. In discussing their health situation, those in this

167

segment think doctors exaggerate how serious a health condition is. Not only is what doctors say unreliable, Resentful Compliers think their doctor would give them an unnecessary prescription drug. At the same time, Resentful Compliers find it difficult to communicate with doctors honestly about their health.

While getting a second opinion is definitely something Resentful Compliers would do, they wouldn't trust the advice of a specialist over that of a general practitioner.

The lack of trust in their doctors is compounded by the Resentful Compliers' difficulty in believing they have a health problem if they cannot see or feel its symptoms. If a Resentful Complier were diagnosed with a disease such as high cholesterol, osteoporosis, or diabetes, he or she may very well reject the diagnosis, considering the physician to be exaggerating or misrepresenting the condition. If prescribed a medication for such so-called symptomless conditions, Resentful Compliers would probably think it unnecessary.

It isn't surprising then that Resentful Compliers admit they do not follow their doctor's instructions. Their conflict and resentment is evident as they question and distrust their doctors' instructions, a situation ripe for the creation of noncompliance. While making their own seemingly uninformed decisions on health, those in this segment still shift responsibility for these decisions to their doctor, the final decision maker.

Open to prescription drugs

It wouldn't bother the Resentful Compliers to know they have to take a prescription drug for as long as they live, nor would they resent taking a prescription drug.

Generally compliant

Resentful Compliers deny they would alter the dos-

168

age on a prescription drug they were taking. Only serious side effects would prompt them to stop taking a prescription drug.

Committed to branded drugs

Direct-to-consumer advertising of pharmaceutical drugs works with Resentful Compliers. Unconvinced their doctor is aware of the best treatments or drugs, Resentful Compliers help their doctor stay informed by taking him or her advertisements for prescription drugs. They are the only Health Compliance segment with this motivation for doing so.

The value of a brand is not lost on Resentful Compliers. Once those in this segment find a brand of a specific prescription drug they believe works for them, they would resent being switched to another. Resentful Compliers are also the only segment that believes branded drugs are better than generic ones. In fact, they trust some manufacturers of branded drugs more than others.

Bothered by high costs, side effects

While rejecting generics and seeking branded prescription drug, Resentful Compliers are also ferociously resentful about the cost of taking prescription drug. Paying for prescription medication presents Resentful Compliers with a serious financial burden. This situation represents another double-bind in which those in this segment find themselves.

Drug interactions and the long-term side-effects of various medications also trouble Resentful Compliers. But even with these very serious concerns, Resentful Compliers wouldn't be willing to try other alternatives, such as lifestyle changes, before starting a prescription drug.

The shape of some pills bothers the Resentful Compliers, and they find them difficult to swallow.

169

Minor involvement with health

Those in this segment are willing to check their body for disease, but they don't appear willing to do much more. Whatever health problems they have, Resentful Compliers don't believe they created them and aren't ready to solve them on their own, as are the Informed Avoiders.

Isolated from their doctors, it's probably beneficial that Resentful Compliers feel comfortable discussing their health problems with interested family and friends. They are also open to reviewing materials from a pharmaceutical manufacturer that would help them to better understand their health conditions and diseases. In addition, Resentful Compliers view their pharmacist as a source of insights on various prescription drugs.

COST-CONCERNED CYNICS

Burdened by the high cost of prescription drugs, Cost-concerned Cynics are angry they must pay for them. If they can, they will choose generics. While they would like to think they are in charge of their health care, other factors, such as their disinterest in becoming informed patients, conflict with this position. Marginally compliant, those in this segment do little to increase their knowledge about their conditions or diseases. Cost-concerned Cynics believe their doctors care about them.

Driven by costs

If given a choice between two prescription drugs, Cost-concerned Cynics will choose the least expensive option. Those in this segment are completely convinced that prescription generic drugs are every bit as good as branded drugs.

Paying for the cost of prescription drugs imposes a serious financial burden on Cost-concerned Cynics. They,

170

like the Resentful Compliers, are angry the costs of pre-scription drugs are so high. As a cost-saving measure, those in this segment would break pills apart and take a partial dose.

A strained relationship

One reason frugal Cost-concerned Cynics follow their doctor's advice is because they have paid for it. Those in this segment also believe their doctors have a genuine concern for them. It doesn't take a long-term relationship with a doctor for Cost-concerned Cynics to develop trust in him or her. While Cost-concerned Cynics would like to believe, they—not their doctor—are the final decision makers on issues impacting their health, this segment lacks the power of information and the financial resources to take charge.

Cost-concerned Cynics have absolutely no expectation that their doctors will deliver certain knowledge regarding their health problems. Nor would Cost-concerned Cynics give greater weight to the advice of a specialist over that of a general practitioner.

Not well informed

While it is difficult for those in this segment to believe they have a disease if they do not feel or see its symptoms, Cost-concerned Cynics don't want to research their medical problems and do not consider it important to do so. Nor do they need to know the details about any illness they may have or understand exactly how a prescription drug they take will resolve their health problem.

While favoring lower-cost, generic drugs, Cost-concerned Cynics also consider DTC advertising as a source of information about how prescription drugs can help them. In addition, those in this segment turn to their pharmacist for information about the prescription drugs they take.

171

Acceptance of prescription drugs

Cost-concerned Cynics wouldn't object to going on a medication, even if it was for the rest of their lives. Doing other things, such as making lifestyle changes, are not realistic options for those in this segment. They prefer to take a prescription drug for a health condition.

Exhibiting marginal compliance

Even after experiencing serious side effects, Cost-concerned Cynics don't think a patient should decide to stop taking a medication. In several other ways, however, Cost-concerned Cynics show they are non-compliant. Not only would they take partial doses to save money, those in this segment don't see a problem with taking a prescription drug on an occasional basis—when they think they need it.

Problems with shape, packaging

Although most affected by concerns over cost, Cost-concerned Cynics also complain that prescription drug containers are difficult to open. For those in this segment, the shape of certain pills makes them difficult to swallow.

PART 4

Chapter 17

EXPLORING SEGMENTS, DIMENSIONS

Evolved from same data

The seven critical health dimensions that make up the Morgan-Levy Health Cube, as well as the three health-related segmentations, Health, Health Compliance, and Health Information, evolved from the same data. Various techniques were applied at different stages of our analysis in order to create our three segmentations, as well as our seven critical dimensions.

Initially, our three health segmentations strategies were created by grouping people with the same or similar responses to hundreds of attitude statements. The statements that most successfully categorized respondents into our segmentations were then analyzed in order to create our seven critical dimensions. Our dimensions represent both a synthesis of our data, as well as a perspective that differs from our segmentation analysis.

Giving dimensions greater depth

Each of the segments resulting from our analysis illustrates the primary ways in which our seven critical

174

dimensions are grouped in the 40 and older U.S. population. In this chapter we examine which dimensions dominate each segment. This perspective provides a better understanding of the seven critical dimensions in the Morgan-Levy Health Cube and also gives each dimension greater depth.

A dual perspective

By looking at both our dimensions and our health-related segments, persons can be viewed in two contexts: single attitude dimensions, such as Concerned over Cost, as well as segments or groups which combine various dimensions, such as the Proactives.

While the dimensions are the primary units of the Morgan-Levy Health Cube, an easy-to-use Internet-based system, the segments in which they appear provide additional background. Each segment has high, average, or low scores on each dimension. It is important to note that these scores are standardized to the normal statistical distribution curve. This means that the score on one dimension can be compared to the score on another dimension, across any segment.

Understanding the scores

The bars in the graphics included in this chapter present each segment's average score on the standard normal distribution for a particular dimension. Some bars are dramatically higher than others: the Trusting Believers' positive score on the Trust in Doctors dimension seen in Figure 17-2 or the Uninvolved Fatalists' negative score on the Healthy Lifestyle dimension shown in Figure 17-1. In these and similar instances the differences are quite obvious.

Other bars are quite short. These short bars are close to or on the zero line and represent an average score. A segment's average score is what one would

175

expect without knowing anything about a segment or person. Longer bars show the relative differences from the average. Whether positive or negative, higher scores, as illustrated by the long bars in the graphics, represent a segment's extreme position on a dimension.

It is immediately apparent that the Proactives' high score on the Healthy Lifestyle dimension is dramatically higher than the Faithful Patients' very low score on this dimension, both shown in Figure 17-1. But it is also important to recognize that while the Confused Compliants segment has an average score on the Healthy Lifestyle dimension, it is still far higher than the Uninvolved Fatalists' very negative score on the same dimension.

Similar scores, differing motivations

One should keep in mind that while two segments may have high scores on a dimension, for instance the Seeks Health-related Information dimension, the motivation behind their high scores may be radically different. To understand the context for their motivations, we turn to the segments.

HEALTHY LIFESTYLE

Three segments have the highest scores on the Healthy Lifestyle dimension: Proactives from our Health segmentation and Internal Health Actives and External Health Actives from our Health Information segmentation. The attitudes of these three segments on the Healthy Lifestyle dimension show they see themselves as highly committed to behaviors supporting a healthful lifestyle.

In contrast, three segments are dramatically negative on this dimension: Faithful Patients from the Health segmentation and Uninvolved Fatalists and

Fearful Listeners from the Health Information segmentation. While all three segments don't see themselves as committed to living a healthy lifestyle, each takes this position for different reasons.

HEALTHY LIFESTYLE SEGMENTS' AVERAGE SCORES

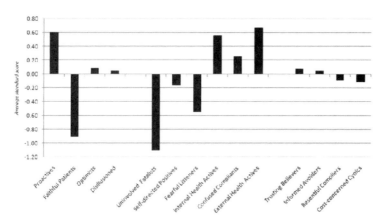

Figure 17-1: *While three segments have high scores on the Healthy Lifestyle dimension, an equal number have exceptionally low scores. For example, Faithful Patients, who know what to do to be healthy, avoid acting on their knowledge. In contrast, Internal Health Actives take responsibility for maintaining good health.*

Faithful Patients know what they should do to stay healthy, but don't follow through. Compared to others in the U.S. population who are 40 and older, those in this segment believe if they become sick, doctors and medications will cure them. Uninvolved Fatalists don't see the point of healthful living because they don't think it will do any good. They are convinced that fate determines their level of health: there is no benefit to living a healthful lifestyle. Distraught by what they see as their current poor health, Fearful Listeners still aren't motivated to act to improve their health. Unfortunately, their procrastination is paired with a willingness to engage in activities having a negative impact on their health.

TRUST IN DOCTORS

Only the Trusting Believers in the Health Compliance segmentation have a very high score on the Trust in Doctors dimension. Those in this segment have a complete belief in their doctors, whom they see as having their best interests at heart. In terms of behavior, we can expect members of this segment to be compliant patients, following their doctors' instructions completely.

Because of their implicit faith in doctors, Trusting Believers shift some—if not most—of the responsibility for their health care to their doctor. Those in this segment have an unshakable belief in their doctors and in the medications they prescribe.

Doctors don't understand

In contrast, Resentful Compliers, also from the Health Compliance segmentation, are extremely negative on the Trust in Doctors dimension. Resentful Compliers have concluded that doctors are not to be trusted. They believe doctors exaggerate the seriousness of a condition and hand out unnecessary prescriptions. Resentful Compliers are convinced their doctors simply don't understand their health problems as well as do they themselves. Compared to those 40 and older, Resentful Compliers believe their doctors don't listen to them and don't really care about them as people. Because of this, Resentful Compliers would not feel compelled to follow a doctor's instructions.

The Disillusioned in our Health segmentation also

have a low score on this dimension. The Disillusioned's negative feelings about doctors are linked to their highly critical views of what they see as our wasteful health-care system. Besides not knowing enough about the interactions of various medications, Disillusioned also fault doctors for not listening to them.

Knowing that someone has scored low on this dimension means he or she should be monitored to make sure medications are being taken and that necessary tests have been performed. In short, a negative score on this dimension is a red flag. For those with negative

TRUST IN DOCTORS
SEGMENTS' AVERAGE SCORES

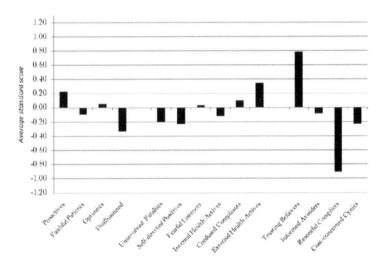

Figure 17-2: *The Trusting Believers' very high score on the Trust in Doctors dimension underscores this segment's total and complete belief in their doctors. In contrast, Resentful Compliers have a number of issues with doctors, including a belief their doctors don't understand their health problems.*

179

scores on the Trust in Doctors dimension nothing could move them to consider their doctor in a favorable light. Viewing their doctors with suspicion and distrust may very well have a negative impact on low scorers' health.

ABLE TO UNDERSTAND HEALTH INFORMATION

Internal Health Actives from our Health Information segmentation have a very high score on this dimension, the highest of all the segments. Internal Health Actives, confident they can assimilate and understand health-related information, act on such information with assurance. A testimonial to the Internal Health Actives' ability to understand health information is their belief that friends and family view them as sources of health information.

A tool for health

Positive scores on this dimension are also seen in the External Health Actives, also in the Health Information segmentation, and the Informed Avoiders from our Health Compliance segmentation. Those in these segments believe they can assimilate and comprehend health information. External Health Actives feel a need to stay healthy in order to care for their families. The information they absorb and understand is a tool to help them achieve this objective. For Informed Avoiders, gathering health-related information allows them to manage and control decisions related to their health.

Because these three segments believe they are able to understand health information, it is possible information directed to them could be more complex or sophisticated than messages made available to those with average or negative scores.

180

ABLE TO UNDERSTAND
HEALTH INFORMATION
SEGMENTS' AVERAGE SCORES

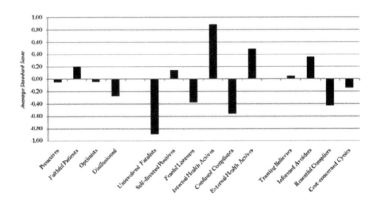

Figure 17-3: *Uninvolved Fatalists see themselves as unable to understand health information. Believing they cannot impact the state of their health, this inability probably does not concern them. In contrast, only Internal Health Actives believe they are viewed as knowledgeable about health information by friends and family.*

Baffled by health information

In contrast, Uninvolved Fatalists, Fearful Listeners, and Confused Compliants from our Health Information segmentation and Resentful Compliers from our Health Compliance segmentation are negative on the Able to Understand Health Information dimension. They believe they are unable to understand health information, which could include instruction from their doctor, inserts provided with prescription drugs, or information about a disease or condition in the New York *Times*.

While those in these four segments believe they are unable to comprehend health-related information, the reasons for this position can include an actual inability to assimilate the material as well as emotional barriers that are obstacles to comprehension.

For example, Uninvolved Fatalists view health information as useless; such information has no value to them. Because of their fatalistic position regarding their health, they are perhaps unwilling to even try to understand health messages. The Fearful Listeners' pessimism about their own health may block their ability to understand health information.

SEEKS HEALTH-RELATED INFORMATION

Two segments within the Health segmentation, the Disillusioned and Faithful Patients, see themselves as motivated on the Seeks Health-related Information dimension. In the Health Information segmentation both Fearful Listeners and External Health Actives have high scores on this dimension. Only the Informed Avoiders in the Health Compliance segmentation score high on believing they are committed to seeking such information.

Information, but no action

While these segments differ on the specific reasons for seeking health-related information, they are all distinguished by the fact that they are intensely convinced they do so at a high or very high level. Faithful Patients, we believe, seek health-related information because it makes them feel they are doing something about their health. This activity could parallel those who collect recipes, but never actually make them. While Faithful Patients collect health-related information, they don't act on it.

Dramatic differences

External Health Actives see health information as a way to stay healthy for those who depend on them, while Informed Avoiders collect the information they need to make informed health-care decisions. Pessimistic about their current state of health, Fearful Listeners are constantly gathering health-related information. But even while seeking information on health, Fearful Listeners are unwilling to try new strategies or make changes to improve their health.

Of the four segments negative on this dimension, the Optimists are the most outstandingly so. It should

SEEKS HEALTH-RELATED INFORMATION
SEGMENTS' AVERAGE SCORES

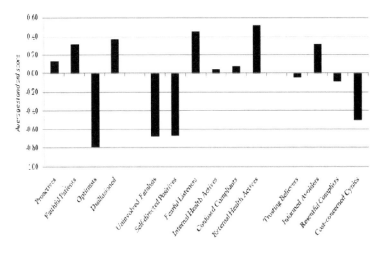

Figure 17-4: Believing they do all that can be done to maintain what they believe is their superb health, Optimists have little interest in seeking health-related information. In contrast, Fearful Listeners, who regard themselves as in poor health, are on a constant quest for additional information.

183

be remembered that Optimists believe they are in good health now and look forward to a healthy future. Convinced they are already doing what is necessary to take care of their health, they apparently see no need to seek health information.

Overwhelmed by costs

Also negative on this dimension are the Cost-concerned Cynics. Their overwhelming concern is over the cost of health care. They may very well believe they don't have the resources to access health information or to follow through on the advice they would receive. In addition, this segment, distrustful of the medical establishment, probably has a jaded view of the benefits of seeking health-related information.

Two segments from the Health Information segmentation are also negative on this dimension: Uninvolved Fatalists and Self-directed Positives. In the case of the latter segment, Self-directed Positives believe they have sufficient information on which to make health decisions. They see no need to pursue additional sources. For Uninvolved Fatalists, fate will determine their health, not insights from health-related information.

SELF-DETERMINATION

Only two segments in our three health-related segmentations have very high scores on this dimension: Optimists in our Health segmentation strategy and Informed Avoiders in our Health Compliance segmentation. Those in both segments wish to retain the locus of control over their health-care decisions. Optimists, as we have pointed out, feel they are very healthy now and don't see that they need outside support; they are in charge.

184

We've mentioned the Informed Avoiders' desire to avoid taking prescription medications and their determination to collect a great deal of health-related information. By amassing such information, the Informed Avoiders are able to retain primary control of their care.

Who is responsible for health?

As previously noted, Trusting Believers in our Health Compliance segmentation strategy have transferred responsibility for their health to their doctors. While Cost-concerned Cynics say they wish to retain control over their health-care decisions, their almost overwhelming concern over health-care costs, as well as their lack of interest in becoming informed patients,

SELF-DETERMINATION
SEGMENTS' AVERAGE SCORES

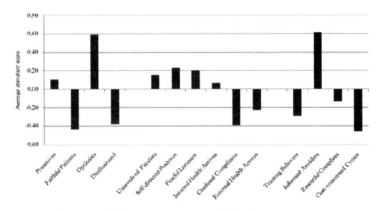

Figure 17-5: High scores on the Self-determination dimension indicate that both Optimists and Informed Avoiders believe they have retained the locus of control over their health-care decisions. Although their reasons differ, segments such as the Confused Compliants and Disillusioned don't see themselves as in charge of their health.

185

conflicts with this desire. The Disillusioned and Faithful Patients from our Health segments also have negative scores on this dimension.

The Disillusioned's low score on the Self-determination dimension is not surprising. Lacking in health insurance, cynical about the medical system, and negative about their doctors, the Disillusioned do not view themselves as in control of their health care. While Faithful Patients are concerned about their health and knowledgeable about what they should do to improve it, they don't take responsibility for it.

Lack of confidence

Confused Compliants in our Health Information strategy are also negative on this dimension. Those in this segment don't see themselves as very smart and lack confidence that they can handle a health crisis. They rely on their doctor's insights and direction.

CONCERNED OVER COST

Only the Disillusioned in the Health segmentation strategy and the Cost-concerned Cynics from the Compliance segmentation score high on this dimension. For their part, the Disillusioned's concern over the cost of health care is understandable. While Disillusioned don't believe they have sufficient health insurance to handle a health-care crisis, they also see an inefficient health-care system as a factor in their lack of access. Those in this segment are committed to the government's providing health insurance to all citizens.

The fear and cynicism felt by the Disillusioned contrasts with the anger flowing from the Cost-concerned Cynics. What they believe to be the high cost of prescription drugs has led them to turn to generics and the

186

practice of taking partial doses.

DTC advertising succeeds

Resentful Compliers are negative on the Concerned over Cost dimension. Their lack of concern over the cost of health care is seen in their attitudes toward drugs. Direct to consumer (DTC) advertising has worked on this segment. Resentful Compliers are convinced branded pharmaceutical drugs are better than generic ones. The cost difference between these two types of pharmaceuticals does not appear to concern them. And they aren't bothered by the idea of continuing to take a prescription drug for the rest of their lives.

CONCERNED OVER COST
SEGMENTS' AVERAGE SCORES

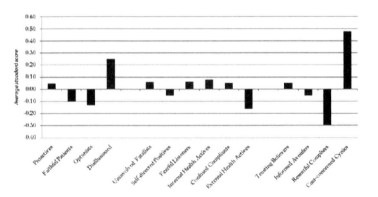

Figure 17-6: Only the Disillusioned and Cost-concerned Cynics see themselves as very concerned over the cost of health care. Resentful Compliers are not bothered by these costs. For example, they prefer branded drugs over generics.

GETTING A CHECKUP

The greatest commitment on the dimension of Getting a Checkup is seen among Proactives. Those in this segment

187

are determined to stay as healthy as possible. The actions they take now, they believe, will determine their future health.

Also scoring high on the Getting a Checkup dimension are the Internal Health Actives, a Health Information segment. Committed to staying in good health, Internal Health Actives see checkups and doctor visits as essential.

In contrast, the Disillusioned have an extremely negative score on this dimension. They feel they have little ability to pay for such doctor visits and because of their cynical view of the medical profession, they may see little value in them.

Convinced of good health

Optimists, also a Health segment, lack interest in seeing a doctor. Believing they are now in very good health and rarely sick, Optimists evidently see little

GETTING A CHECKUP
SEGMENTS' AVERAGE SCORES

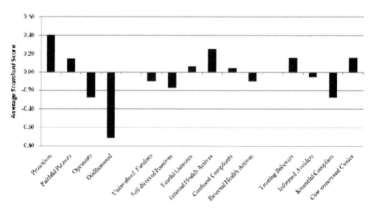

Figure 17-7: The greatest commitment to getting checkups is found among Proactives who believe doctor visits will help them stay healthy. Lacking access, as well as having a critical view of the practice of health care, Disillusioned have a negative perspective of such visits.

188

reason to maintain regular checkups with their doctor. But the good health Optimists believe they have may very well be based on some false assumptions. Because they avoid going to the doctor for checkups or visits, they have little objective proof of good health. Optimists also question the value of such visits. If they were to get sick, Optimists don't believe there was anything they could have done to prevent the illness.

Resentful Compliers, a Health Compliance segment, also see little value in checkups as evidenced by their somewhat low score on this dimension. Those in this segment see little benefit from a doctor visit; they don't view doctors as authoritative sources for guidance in health matters. One example of the Resentful Compliers' profound lack of trust in their doctors is their belief that doctors tend to overstate health concerns. Why visit a doctor who, in their view, lies, exaggerates, and is ill informed?

Chapter 18

USING THE MORGAN-LEVY HEALTH CUBE

Three ways to use

Data from the Morgan-Levy Health Cube can be used in three fundamental ways. Those completing it can use the information for themselves and keep the results private. If they wish, the results can also be shared on a person-to-person basis, whether the relationship is as a patient, employee, insured, or simply an interested party.

In the third use of the Morgan-Levy Health Cube's insights, data are compiled into a database and used to understand the health-care motivations of large populations. These populations could be employees, takers of a pharmaceutical drug, or subscribers to a health-related magazine.

Gathering data

Patients, employees, and others complete the Morgan-Levy Health Cube on a computer, after using a personal identification code to access our website. Assured of confidentiality, persons completing our system

190

decide if they wish to share their information with their doctor, a wellness coach, their employer, a government entity, or a marketing organization.

After answering a series of defining questions, the individual instantly receives a report based on his or her score on the seven critical dimensions. The report gives the participant's scores against the average score for the 40 and older U.S. population on that dimension. The report also outlines the scores' implications and contains suggestions for potential next steps. The participant may decide to act in order to increase or decrease his or her score on one or more dimensions.

Interest in feedback

For a number of reasons, we believe Americans are highly motivated to take the Morgan-Levy Health Cube. Most of us are naturally curious; we want to learn more about why we act as we do.

Americans have a long history of taking part in all types of self-assessment tests. As teenagers, we may have completed a *Glamour* magazine quiz on what constitutes a dream date. Completing an IQ test on the Mensa web site or career assessments and aptitude tests may have followed. Taking such tests is natural for us.

We also have a culture of self-improvement and self-help. Many of us would like to improve how we do things. New insights resulting from the self-tests we take or those administered by professionals, such as the Myers-Briggs, give us insights from which we believe we can benefit. Some of the tests we take also hold out the promise of an economic benefit.

The Morgan-Levy Health Cube provides individuals with unique information on the attitudes and motivations underlying their health-related choices. Knowing their scores on the seven critical dimensions, persons can decide whether or not they wish to change attitudes which may be impediments to their good health. Research shows that once attitudes are altered, a change in behaviors often follows. Rather than disorganized or piecemeal attempts to figure out motivations behind potentially damaging choices, the Morgan-Levy Health Cube facilitates working from a comprehensive assessment and focusing energies.

Costs shift to individuals

Besides the enjoyment of better health for its own sake, individuals will also find improving their health has an economic benefit. Over the past decade, individuals receiving health insurance coverage from their employers have seen the cost of such coverage shift to them. In addition, while some employers reward participants in wellness programs, others penalize those who smoke or are overweight by requiring them to pay a larger share of their insurance premiums.

It appears inexorable that the cost of health insurance and care will shift increasingly to individuals, whether employees, retirees, or the self-employed. For employees, this shift may require that they take on the responsibility of securing their own health insurance, perhaps receiving a stipend from their employer in order to do so. We have already witnessed the passing of defined benefit pension plans, largely replaced by 401 (k)s.

Better health rewarded

Under this evolving scenario, those who are in better health will undoubtedly receive more and better health insurance at a lower cost. Today non-smokers benefit from lower premiums than smokers. In the not too distant future, we will have to be savvy buyers of health-care insurance, as well as maintainers of the highest level of health possible. If not, we will suffer physical, emotional, and financial consequences.

As health insurance costs shift, individuals wishing to control their health-care expenditures will have to eat a balanced diet, maintain a normal weight, quit smoking, and exercise regularly. To accomplish these goals, they will have to obtain and use insights on their own health choices, including their attitudes toward specific health dimensions.

Need to assess motivations

Today wellness programs provide feedback on individuals' current health. Assessments of blood sugar levels, exercise, and the ability to deal with stress are all of value in establishing one's current health and potential health risks. These assessments are, however, limited because they are not typically paired with an equally rigorous assessment of an individual's motivations.

If persons do not see the value of a healthy lifestyle, why would they be motivated to change? If persons have little trust in their doctor, why would they follow his or her recommendations? Insights from the Morgan-Levy Health Cube provide individuals with a quick, but reliable, assessment of their motivations on seven critical health-related issues. It will be of great benefit to know if a score on one of the dimensions could be an obstacle to health.

A tool for health professionals

In order to provide better care, avoid medical errors, increase compliance, and improve their patients' health, today's health-care professionals are being asked to improve the way in which they communicate with patients. They are being asked to understand their patients' health-related motivations. While learning communication skills is now part of the curriculum for most health-care providers, it is a somewhat recent development. It was not until 2002 that the Accreditation Council for Graduate Medical Education "required the teaching and assessment of interpersonal and communication skills."[1]

Even with this requirement, teaching communication skills in some residency programs "has received relatively low priority."[2] We believe these courses are still rudimentary. For example, in medical schools most of this instruction takes place within the first two years, when students have far less patient contact than during the final two years.

Some not trained

In addition, one-third of all doctors currently practicing are 55 and older.[3] They have probably never had any training in patient communication skills having completed medical school much before 2002. Unfortunately, after leaving medical school "most physicians never get feedback about their interactions with patients."[4]

The courses health professionals take suggest ways in which they can become good, active listeners. Through role playing, sometimes involving professional actors, health-care professionals increase their focus on patients' needs. They are taught to encourage patients to verbalize by nodding in agreement as they speak. These professionals are instructed to be patient and take the time to listen. But, as we have mentioned elsewhere in this book, the average doctor visit currently lasts 22 minutes.

In practicing patient-centered communications, "Physicians need to perform multiple communication tasks during interactions with patients."[5] It seems doubtful a health-care professional has the time or skills to extract relevant information regarding the individual patient's concerns, needs, motivations, and values and then translate those into an effective response all within a few minutes. While it is true that today health-care professionals are taught basic communication skills, it remains difficult for these efforts to result in deep insights into a patient's values and motivations.

Individuals, not groups

And while health professionals may be taught how to communicate with a specific type of patient, the instruction often addresses the patient as a member of a group, such as Hispanics or the elderly. This application, then, focuses on a broad class and not on the underlying motivations of an individual patient. This approach is, in our view, too general to be very useful. We don't accept the idea that all Hispanics have the same values or that all persons over 65 share the same motivations.

Patients themselves constrained

The question also remains whether or not the patient can articulate concerns, needs and wishes. Do patients have the self-awareness and assertiveness to pinpoint their needs in the few minutes spent with a doctor or nurse? For example, can obese patients discern the motivations which keep them from loosing weight and communicate them? Does the patient trust the health-care provider sufficiently to reveal these issues? Or are patients so distrustful they aren't receptive to anything a doctor, dentist, or nurse might say?

The results of the Morgan-Levy Health Cube complement any training a health professional has had. This information enables a doctor or wellness counselor to move to a deeper level of communication. A patient or employee, for example, can be counseled by a pharmacist, doctor, or wellness professional using insights generated by our system.

Putting it into practice

Knowing that a patient has a high score on the Healthy Lifestyle dimension would guide a physician or a wellness counselor to ask questions and make recommendations that would be far different than those asked without this information. With these insights from the Morgan-Levy Health Cube, it would not be necessary to waste time trying to convince the patient of the benefits of a healthy lifestyle. Instead, the doctor or wellness counselor could begin a discussion with the specific steps the patient can take to realize his or her own motivations.

Body language and statements of assurance and concern might be more frequent and the language more supportive after noting a patient has an extremely low score on the Trust in Doctors dimension. Knowing that a patient has a low score on the Seeks Health-related Information dimension should temper the amount of health-related information handed out by a health professional, such as a wellness counselor.

A doctor should address the concerns of patients with high scores on the Concerned over Cost dimension. Do these patients split pills or skip doses, thereby reducing their dosage—or not fill a prescription altogether? At this point, the doctor could also discuss generics, samples, and pharmaceutical programs.

Applied one-on-one, insights from the Morgan-Levy Health Cube can help the health-care professional tailor messages, select body language, gauge the amount and complexity of information to dispense, and structure treatment and wellness plans reflecting the person's own motivations.

Database applications

With assurances for the protection of each individual's identity and privacy and with the respondent's permission, individual responses from the Morgan-Levy Health Cube can be used to build a database, whether of patients in a practice, users or potential users of a prescription drug, or members of a health-care plan. Potentially all Medicare recipients or employees 40 and older could take the Morgan-Levy Health Cube and receive their scores and reports.

Individual categorizations could form a database of scores on our seven critical health dimensions and our segments. This data could then be cross-referenced with behaviors, such as levels of exercise, and demographics, such as age and income, as well as diseases and conditions.

Insights for Medicare

Wide-ranging use of the Morgan-Levy Health Cube could give the Department of Health and Human Services the ability to examine those on Medicare not only by utilization and diseases, but also by health-related motivations.

Kerry Weems, Acting Administrator of the Centers for Medicare & Medicaid Services (CMS), has expressed interest in finding ways "to help Medicare beneficiaries identify their health risks . . . and provide them with information and support they need to proactively take better care of their health." [6]

To that end, Medicare funded demonstration projects attempting to determine whether employee wellness programs could be adapted to its population and be effective in delaying the onset of chronic disease.

In a paper published in *Clinical Interventions in Aging*, the authors conclude that "A growing literature presents convincing evidence that seniors who reduce

197

their modifiable health risks can forestall disability, reduce their utilization of health services, and ultimately
save Medicare money."[7] Some suggest that beginning
such preventive efforts prior to Medicare enrollment
could have long-term benefits.

For example, an article in *Health Affairs* suggests
that making a weight-loss program available to persons
with pre-diabetes who are 60 to 64 could generate lifetime savings of $7 billion or more for Medicare. The
parameters employed in the authors' calculations includes a participation rate of 55 percent, a rate
"typically reported in well-designed workplace wellness programs."[8]

Are nonparticipants forgotten?

While it is gratifying that more than half of those
eligible for this weight-loss program are projected to
participate in it, what of the other 45 percent? What
attitudes and motivations keep them from participating
in the program? Are those who elect to enroll in the
program already convinced of the benefits of a healthful lifestyle and now ready to take action?

It seems obvious that we must understand the non-
participation of 45 percent of this and other populations. The Morgan-Levy Health Cube provides perspectives on attitudes which keep some individuals
from taking part in wellness programs. In addition, it
identifies those attitudes which need to be reinforced
among those already motivated to participate.

Tailored messages, programs needed

Insights from the Morgan-Levy Health Cube can
contribute to the success of preventive programs by tai-
loring individual communications, and the programs
themselves, to the individual, based on his or her needs
and interests. It is important to note that a RAND study

found that successful risk reduction programs "employ tailored and personalized interventions . . . "[9] Weems has stated Medicare's interest in providing "tailored information and support to beneficiaries."[10]

The completion of the Morgan-Levy Health Cube by Medicare recipients would add the critical motivational perspective to data on demographics, behaviors, and health status. An understanding of the all-important *why*, the motivations underlying someone's avoidance of exercise or high level of compliance, provides insights for truly targeted communication and support.

Measuring change

The use of health-care services is not shaped solely by physicians, but also by patients. As we have described, each patient 40 and older scores somewhere on a continuum on each of the seven critical dimensions. It makes sense to focus different messages and programs on very dissimilar populations. A retaking of the Morgan-Levy Health Cube at a later date, perhaps after a public-health campaign, could measure any movement up or down each dimension.

Employee wellness

In 2010, 74 percent of North American companies offered a employee wellness program.[11] Employees were encouraged to do such things as stop smoking, increase their amount of exercise, loose weight, or improve the way in which they care for a chronic condition, such as diabetes. Such actions will not only improve employees' lives, but reduce their employers' health-care costs. It is estimated that in 2010 employers spent $220 on each employee participating in a wellness program.[12] The return on this investment could be increased by being able to easily and quickly understand the health-related motivations of employees 40 and older.

There are two ways in which an employer and its employees can benefit from the Morgan-Levy Health Cube. If an employee decides to participate in the Morgan-Levy Health Cube system, he or she can log on to our secure site and answer the questions on a computer, whether at home or work. These individual answers and the resulting report are completely confidential.

Working with a counselor

If the employee is working with a wellness or disease management counselor, he or she can decide to share the confidential results. In doing so, the employee will benefit because counselors can then use results from the Health Cube to better focus messages and suggestions directed at the specific employee. Rather than spend precious and costly hours conducting interviews probing to arrive at the employee's motivations, the counselor will instantly know that person's attitudinal profile on seven health-related dimensions.

Large populations classified

With their employees' permission, and assuring the protection of each individual's privacy and identity, data gathered from those who have taken the Morgan-Levy Health Cube can give employers insights into trends within job classes and locations, as well as utilization of health insurance. In this instance, individual employees are not identified.

Through an analysis of data gathered from hundreds, if not thousands of employees, employers will know if a certain category of employee scores higher or lower on a particular dimension or if employees working at a particular location have higher or lower scores

200

than others working somewhere else.

Employees working in California, for example, may have higher scores on the Healthy Lifestyle dimension than those in Massachusetts. It may be that more managers have lower scores on the Concerned over Cost dimension than employees at the clerical level.

Employers who have identified groups of employees with similar scores on key dimensions could develop or offer seminars and training targeting shared motivations. For example, those who score low on the Able to Understand Health Information dimension could be offered a seminar structured around suggestions to increase comprehension of health information.

Programs to prevent, manage disease

In the same way in which employers, with their employees permission, can construct large databases and study them to arrive at important conclusions, so too can managed care organizations and health-insurance providers. The benefits of a disease-management program would be enhanced if providers of such services had insights into the population of those with a disease, such as chronic obstructive pulmonary disease (COPD).

The provider of disease management services may find that, as a group, those with COPD score dramatically lower on the Healthy Lifestyle dimension. Rather than deal with other dimensions at that time, the strategic decision could be made to focus on messages and programs communicating the importance of exercise, not smoking, and a healthy diet among this population.

Marketing strategy

Marketers of any health-related service or product, from a cholesterol-reducing drug to a hip implant to a chain of surgical centers, would find it useful to add the Morgan-Levy Health Cube to their market research.

Obtaining such information on a target population would give these marketers a rich and deep background regarding this population's motivations on health.

What portion of the 40 and older population is composed of persons scoring high on the Self-determination dimension, probably seeking to avoid hip or knee replacement therapy, as well as medications? This insight would be relevant to companies ranging from Pfizer to Medtronic.

While specific motivational or attitudinal segmentations are highly useful, for example, one on taking a drug for high cholesterol, such strategies can be crossed with data from the Morgan-Levy Health Cube for an even deeper understanding of a target's motivations.

Marketing communications

Whether for advertising, direct marketing, public relations, or e-marketing, knowing the health-related attitudes of a specific market would be of great help in both positioning a product or service, as well as creating messages appealing to the specific attitudinal composition of the target.

Leo Francis, president of Publicis Medical Education Group, stresses the fact that "Only by understanding . . . most importantly, the perspective through the patients' eyes, can marketers identify and fully respond to the needs of people living with an illness."[13]

"New technologies to map and track individuals' attitudes and behavior will allow us to create the right message with the right tone in the right place at the right time," believes David Davenport-Firth, Global Brand Strategy Director of Ogilvy CommonHealth Worldwide.[14]

Insights from the Morgan-Levy Health Cube can be used to identify and shape messages relevant to a specific individual or audience. We have shown that depending on their score on a particular dimension, individuals prefer specific sources of health-related information. Shaped by our system, tailored messages can be transmitted through a preferred channel, whether in a doctor's office or through social media, using technologies which already exist.

Integrating the platform

Once someone has completed the Morgan-Levy Health Cube and the results have been captured electronically, a platform has been established on which several applications can be built and integrated.

We have suggested that individuals will obtain insights on their own health-related attitudes through the use of our system. Moving from the individual, we note beneficial applications, ranging from employee wellness programs, to the content of health-related information on the Internet, from DTC advertising in magazines, to physicians knowing how their patients' values and attitudes might affect compliance.

The Morgan-Levy Health Cube offers all the ability to weave together a cohesive communication strategy existing on multiple levels.

REFERENCES

[1] Wendy Levinson, et al. "Developing Physician Communication Skills for Patient-Centered Care. Health Affairs 29.7 (2010): 1310-1318. Print.

[2] Levinson, et al.

[3] Robert Davis. "Shortage of surgeons pinches U.S. hospitals." *saynotocaps.org*. USA Today, 26 Feb. 2008. Web. 5 March 2011.

[4] Levinson, et al,

[5] Levinson, et al.

[6] "Medicare Makes Awards for Senior Risk Reduction Demonstration As Part Of Focus on Prevention, USA." Medical News Today, 19 Dec., 2007. Web. 9 Nov. 2011.

[7] Ron Z. Goetzel, et al. "Can health promotion programs save Medicare money?" PubMed Central, March 2007. Web. 7 July 2010.

[8] Kenneth E. Thorpe and Zhou Yang. "Enrolling People With Prediabetes Ages 60-64 In A Proven Weight Loss Program Could Save Medicare $7 Billion Or More." Health Affairs 30.9 (2011): 1673-1679. Print.

[9] Ron Z. Goetzel, et al.

[10] "Medicare Makes Awards for Senior Risk Reduction Demonstration As Part Of Focus on Prevention, USA."

[11] Stephen Miller. "U.S. Businesses Spend More on Wellness Programs, But Most Don't Measure Results." *shrm.org.* Society for Human Resource Management, 1 Oct. 2011. Web. 5 March 2011.

[12] Miller.

[13] Robin Robinson. "Social Media and Patient Education: Where the Patients Are." PharmaVOICE Oct. 2011: 14-20. Print.

[14] David Davenport-Firth. "202020 Vision." PharmaVOICE March 2011: 106-107. Print.

Chapter 19

FOCUS ON THE
INDIVIDUAL

Devouring our economy

For decades, we have observed the health-care avalanche thundering towards us, threatening to overwhelm our economy. For the past 50 years, the cost of health care has steadily increased, more dramatically at times than others. Our expenditures on health care as a percentage of GDP has relentlessly risen with each passing year. In 2020, a mere eight years from now, it is projected that the cost of health care will consume 19.8 percent of our economy.[1] At that time, it is possible that one dollar in five will be spent on health.

A precipitous decline

If health-care costs continue to increase at the current pace, our ability "to pay for nonhealth goods and services—such as education, infrastructure, and consumer goods—will be compromised."[2] In a pair of articles, Michael Chernew, Richard Hirth, and David Cutler conclude that "if health care costs continued to

205

grow at two percentage points per year above real per capita GDP growth, the United States would experience major reductions in the consumption of nonhealth goods and services . . . "[3] Unless "the rate of health cost growth can be lowered," we would begin "a precipitous decline" in 2050.

Individuals key to a cure

Each U.S. citizen 40 and older, the primary consumer of health care today, can contribute significantly to mitigating the impact of the health-care avalanche. Both today and in the future, it is the individual who consumes health care. What type of care the individual uses, as well as how much, is central to our ability to control health-care expenditures. By making more healthful choices, individuals can reduce the incidence of chronic diseases which are today devouring the majority of our health-care dollars.

We recognize the causes for our monumental health-care costs are several and complex. From paperwork requirements to the lack of quality in the services delivered, from the use of unproven, ineffective treatments to a lack of compliance, there are a myriad of issues, each contributing to our high-cost health care. But individual consumption is the trigger that increases use.

Need to know costs

As the health-care avalanche thunders ever closer, various economic and medical changes are taking place. While the majority of health consumers today lack information on the cost of their health care, forces are in play making it imperative for them to become educated as to the true cost of the health care they receive. The need for this type of knowledge is paired with the economic fact that employers, significant providers of health insurance coverage in the U.S., are

206

shifting the cost of such coverage to their employees.

Individuals bear more costs

From 1999 to 2009, for example, employees assumed increasing responsibility for their health-insurance coverage and the care it provides. Over that time period, premiums, deductibles and co-pays all increased. A family of four, for example, saw its monthly premium rise by 128 percent, while its out-of-pocket spending for health care increased by 78 percent.[4]

While it is true that a family of this size with employer-provided health insurance saw a $95 increase in median monthly income from 1999 to 2009, these gains were largely consumed by increased spending on health care. In addition, instead of $95, the increase in monthly income over those ten years would have been $545 if "the rate of health care cost growth had not exceeded general inflation."[5]

And employees and others will continue to pay more for health insurance. For example, a study by the National Business Group on Health shows that in 2012 "53% of employers plan to increase employees' share of premiums, while 39% plan to increase in-network deductibles."[6] Such financial changes make it necessary for employees, or any buyers of health insurance, to become increasingly knowledgeable about what it is they are buying and how they can obtain the best coverage for themselves at the lowest cost.

Working together

At the same time, those who provide health care are becoming increasingly dedicated to the idea of patient-centered care. The patient and his or her doctor are seen as working together to achieve better health. Again, such a development requires a patient aware of his or her needs, who is an articulate communicator, one who can understand the benefits and drawbacks of various health-care options.

Healthful living key

The individual too is at the heart of another shift that lies within our basic perception of the role of medicine in our health care. Some authorities advocate a shift in medicine from the treatment of acute disease to that of prevention. And prevention, whether in the form of public health campaigns or screening examinations, requires the cooperation and commitment of individual persons, each one distinct and different.

Targeted communication needed

In order to achieve a significant measure of involvement in prevention strategies from a person, whether as a patient, purchaser of health insurance, or customer, communication with that person will enjoy the greatest success if it is tailored to motivate him or her.

The developments we have outlined above, as well as others, demand the individual become informed, responsible, and involved in his or her health care. Individuals must recognize not only behavioral or demographic impediments to their good health, but must also have an acute awareness of their attitudes, attitudes that may encourage or block a movement to better health habits.

Reliable, low-cost tool

The Morgan-Levy Health Cube provides a cost-effective and quick way of assessing health-related attitudes of individuals 40 and older in the U.S. population. This knowledge allows for the creation of targeted communications that motivate each person most effectively.

In addition, those who provide health services and products, whether doctors or nurses, those marketing public health programs or pharmaceuticals, or those promoting employee wellness or compliance, will be better able to understand someone's health-related attitudes and what they should say or do to best engage the motivations of this unique individual.

REFERENCES

[1] Sean P. Keehan, et al. "National Health Spending Projections Through 2020: Economic Recovery and Reform Drive Faster Spending Growth." *healthaffairs.org*. Health Affairs 30.8 (2011):1594-1605. Web. 17 Oct. 2011.

[2] Benjamin D. Sommers. "Why Lowering Health Costs Should Be A Key Adjunct to Slowing Health Spending Growth." *healthaffairs.org*. Health Affairs 29.9 (2010):1651-1655. Web. 17 Oct. 2011.

[3] Sommers.

[4] David I. Auerbach and Arthur L. Kellerman. "A Decade of Health Care Cost Growth Has Wiped Out Real Income Gains For An Average US Family." *healthaffairs.org*. Health Affairs 30.9 (2011):1630-1636. Web. 17 Oct. 2011.

[5] Auerbach and Kellerman.

[6] Sandra Block. "Rising health costs get harder to escape." USA Today, 10 Oct. 2011. Print.

APPENDICES

Appendix A

RELIABILITY

Scales

Reliability measures the consistency of a set of measures. Using a set of scales, the same results should occur from one measurement in time to another using the same scale. For example, the usefulness of a bathroom scale is based on our knowledge that if it is working correctly every time we use it the results will be based on consistent measurements.

Our dimensions are based on a set of agree to disagree scales measuring our respondents' attitudes on a number of health issues. Unless influenced by something or someone else, attitudes tend to be persistent. If the retesting of respondents yields similar responses for each health issue, we know the scales we used are reliable.

To test the reliability of our scales, we resurveyed respondents from our 1996, 1997 and 1998 samples in 2004. We intended to determine both the reliability of our scales and confirm our predictions of the segments into which we had originally categorized our respondents.

212

Some criticize the retesting of the same respondents because if the time separating the periods is too short, respondents may remember their answers. Since the time periods between our surveys were at least six years and, at most, eight years apart, that criticism does not apply in this case.

Our Health segmentation was conducted in all four years; our Health Information segmentation in 1997, 1998, and 2004; and our Health Compliance segmentation in 1998 and 2004. Because of these differences, sample sizes varied.

The table below shows the range of correlations and sample sizes for the scales in the three segmentations. "Significance level" refers to the likelihood that we have incorrectly claimed the respondents gave similar scores between the two testing periods. Statistically there is only a one in a thousand chance the two scores each respondent gave us are *not* related. The analysis clearly shows that respondents were consistent in their answers, even though they completed our questionnaires from six- to eight-year intervals.

Segments

We tested the reliability of our segmentations by

Segmentation	Range of correlations	Range of sample sizes	Significance level
Health (1996, 1997, 1998 vs. 2004)	0.30-0.62	1,764-1,779	p <0.001 all scales
Health Information (1997, 1998 vs. 2004)	0.29-0.42	1,108-1,116	p <0.001 all scales
Health Compliance (1998 vs. 2004)	0.26-0.48	514-517	p <0.001 all scales

213

comparing the predicted segment of each respondent in 2004 with the original prediction in either 1996, 1997 or 1998.

This correlation result is statistically significant at a probability of being wrong at less than one in a thousand (p <0.001). Thus, our predictions of a respondent's segment over the six- to eight-year periods measured are reliable. Similar results occurred with our Health Compliance and Health Information segmentations.

Figure A-1 shows our respondents overwhelmingly remained in the same Health segment over time. In each segment, either a majority or plurality of respondents continued to be classified in the same segment in 2004 as in 1996, 1997, and 1998.

PERCENT OF HEALTH SEGMENTS IN 2004

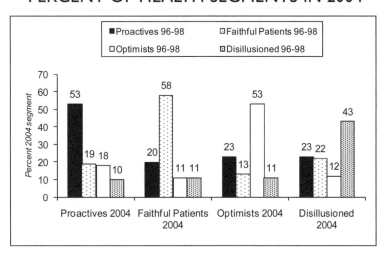

Figure A-1: In each segment, the majority or plurality of respondents continued to be classified in the same segment in 2004 as in 1996, 1997, and 1998.

214

Appendix B

VALIDITY

Our system is based on the premise that a positive change in a person's attitudes about his or her health increases the likelihood that the person will adopt more healthful behaviors.

If this premise is true, implementing programs using insights from our system will lead people to adopt healthier attitudes. The result will be a decrease in medical expenditures and a better quality of life for many participants.

In order to achieve these results, our system must be valid. Validity is the degree to which a test measures what it says it will measure.

To validate our system, we resurveyed 1,800 people across the United States in 2004 whom we had originally randomly surveyed in either 1996, 1997, or 1998. In each of these three years, we had recruited different samples. Since the questionnaires were essentially the same, we were able to combine respondents from the three years, enabling us to work with a larger sample size for this analysis.

The behaviors we chose to examine were: (1) weight control, (2) exercise level, and (3) smoking. Health researchers have overwhelmingly determined that keeping one's weight at a normal level, getting sufficient exercise, and not using tobacco are critical to good health.

Our Health segmentation consists of four segments, but one segment, the Proactives, most consistently practices these healthful behaviors. We predicted that respondents who were not Proactives in 1996-98 *but* who became Proactives in 2004 were more likely to have both adopted proactive attitudes *and* also to have improved in these three critical health behaviors.

Weight control

We asked our respondents in 1997, 1998, and 2004 to tell us their height and weight. These measures were not collected in the 1996 survey. Using these measures, we calculated each respondent's body mass index (BMI). This index is the ratio of metric weight divided

HEALTH SEGMENTS BY
BODY MASS INDEX

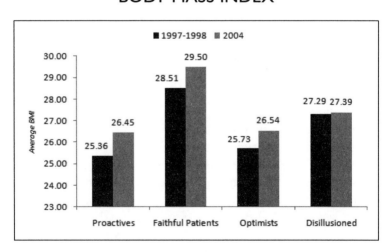

Figure B-1: *In 1996-8 and in 2004, Proactives, along with Optimists, had lower BMI scores than the other two Health segments.*

216

by metric height squared. Having a normal weight, defined by the National Institutes of Health as having a BMI of between 18.5 and 24.9, is optimum.

Figure B-1 on the previous page shows Proactives, along with the Optimists, having a lower BMI than Faithful Patients and Disillusioned in both the combined 1997 and 1998 surveys and in 2004.

Figure B-2 shows the change in BMI among those who were *not* Proactives in 1997-8. This figure compares the change in BMI of those who adopted Proactives' attitudes in 2004 versus those who did not. The chart shows the *average difference* between each person's BMI in 1997-8 as compared to their BMI in 2004.

On average, those who became Proactives increased their BMI by 0.22 points. In contrast, those

CHANGE IN BODY MASS INDEX
AMONG EARLIER NON-PROACTIVES

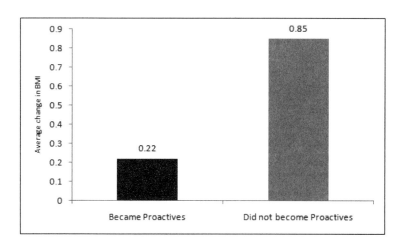

Figure B-2: *This chart shows the average change in BMI by those non-Proactives in 1997-8. Those who became Proactives in 2004 had gained significantly less weight than those who did not become Proactives.*

217

who did not become Proactives increased their BMI by 0.85 points. Those respondents who did not become Proactives in 2004 had an almost a four-fold increase in BMI over those who became Proactives. This change is statistically significant (p <0.01).

Exercise level

To measure exercise behavior, we were precise about its intensity, as well as its frequency. We asked each respondent "how many times a week do you exercise within the range of your target heart rate? That is, so that you feel as if you are working hard for at least 20 minutes each time and are to the point that you might be a bit short of breath or feel your heart is

HEALTH SEGMENTS
AEROBIC EXERCISE
ONCE A WEEK OR MORE

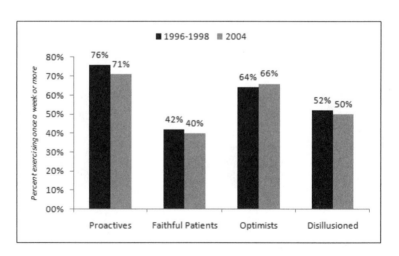

Figure B-3: In 1996-8 and in 2004, Proactives and Optimists had the highest percentage of persons who exercised aerobically once a week or more.

218

pounding harder?"

A total of 1,778 people age 40 and older answered this exercise question in the period 1996-8 and once again in 2004.

Figure B-3 shows that Proactives and Optimists had the highest percentages of those who exercised aerobically once a week or more.

Figure B-4 examines the 1,211 people who were *not* Proactives in 1996-8. We predicted persons who would be classified as Proactives in 2004 would have a greater proportion of exercisers than those who were not classified as Proactives. As the graph shows, new Proactives outnumber non-Proactives and at a statistically significant level (p <0.001).

PROPORTION EXERCISING IN 2004 AMONG EARLIER NON-PROACTIVES

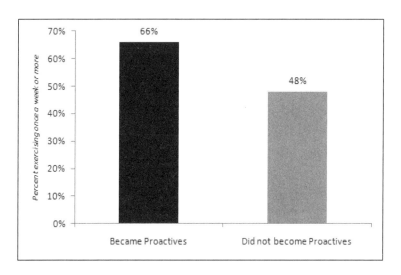

Figure B-4: Those not classified as Proactives in 1996-8 who were later classified as Proactives in 2004 have a statistically higher proportion of exercisers as compared to those not classified in 2004 as Proactives.

Smoking

The third behavior of interest to us was smoking. In 1996-8, we asked "what is your use of cigarettes, cigars or pipes?" The respondents were given the choice of "currently use," "used in past," or "never used." We hypothesized that fewer of those respondents who were Proactives would smoke as compared to those who were not Proactives. Secondly, we believed that fewer of those who became Proactives in 2004 would smoke as compared to those who did not become Proactives.

Figure B-5 shows that in both the 1996-8 time period as well as in 2004, Proactives had the lowest percentage of smokers.

Figure B-6 shows that, as predicted, the incidence of smoking in 2004 was lower among those who were non-Proactives in 1996-8, but who became Proactives in 2004, as compared to those who did not adopt the Proactives' mindset ($p<0.01$).

HEALTH SEGMENTS
PERCENT SMOKERS

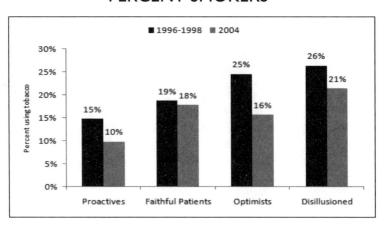

Figure B-5: *In both periods, Proactives had the lowest percent of those smoking.*

220

PROPORTION OF SMOKERS
AMONG EARLIER NON-PROACTIVES

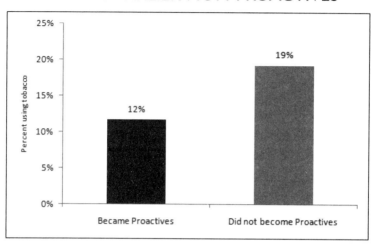

Figure B-6: Of those non-Proactives in 1996-8, significantly fewer smokers are found among those who became Proactives in 2004, than those who did not change to this segment.

Conclusions on validity

On each of three critical health-related behaviors, we have shown statistically significant increases in healthful behaviors among those who became Proactives.

We conclude that persons can change motivational segments. In addition, we have shown that changes in attitudes are mirrored to a significant degree in changes in behavior. Having made these positive changes, these newly minted Proactives will enjoy better health and incur lower medical expenses.

221

INDEX OF SUBJECTS

C

Caffeine, *see* Food components
Calories, *see* Food components
Cancer, *see* Diseases
Centers for Disease Control and Prevention (CDC), 48-49,
    64-67, 115
Children in household, *see* Demographics
Cholesterol, *see* Food components
Cholesterol, *see* Preventive tests
Chronic diseases, multiple, 43, 60-61, 77-78, 88, 98, 112-13,
    124
Cold medications, *see* Drugs, Over-the-counter (OTC)
Congestive heart failure, *see* Diseases
Cost of health care, 2, 9, 29, 121, 127, 130, 184, 186-87,
    205
Cough syrup, *see* Drugs, Over-the-counter (OTC)

D

Death, 48-49, 66-67, 129
Demographics
    Children in household, 38, 59, 74, 85, 95, 109, 122
    Gender, 24, 38, 74, 85, 95
    Income, 24, 38, 48, 59, 74, 85, 95, 108, 122, 127, 197,
        207
    Marital status, 38, 59, 74, 95, 109, 122
    Educational level,   48, 74, 85, 95, 108-09, 112
Depression, *see* Diseases
Diabetes, *see* Diseases
Diet pills, *see* Drugs, Over-the-counter (OTC)
Dimensions
    Able to Understand Health Information, 3, 36, 107-19,
        180-82, 201
    Concerned over Cost, 34, 36, 121-30, 175, 187, 196,
        201

Health maintenance organization (HMO),
    see Health Insurance
Hospital visits, 9, 46, 50, 76, 112, 116-118, 129-130
    Inpatient, 40, 61,67, 75, 86, 97, 112, 124
    Outpatient, 61, 86, 97, 124

I

Income, *see* Demographics
Insurance *see* Health insurance
Internet, 27, 29, 45, 79, 101-03, 114, 126, 203
    see also Health communication sources

L

Laxatives, *see* Drugs, Over-the-counter (OTC)
Lifestyles, 11, 38, 46, 53

M

Magazines, *see* Health communication sources
Major medical, *see* Health insurance
Males, *see* Demographics, Gender
Mammogram, *see* Preventive tests
Marital status, *see* Demographics
Marketing, 6, 28, 201-02, 209
Medicaid, *see* Health Insurance
Medicare, *see* Health Insurance
Migraines, *see* Diseases
Morgan-Levy Health Cube, 3-6, 20-22, 24-25, 27, 29, 31, 34
    -35, 43, 134-36, 174-75, 190-203, 208
Multiple chronic diseases, 43, 60, 77, 88, 98, 112, 124

N

Newsletters, *see* Health communication sources
Newspapers, *see* Health communication sources

No health insurance, *see* Health Insurance
Non-health-related magazines, *see* Health communication
    sources
Nurse, *see* Health communication sources

O

Obesity; overweight, 50-53, 192
Osteoporosis, *see* Diseases

P

Paid health newsletters, *see* Health communication sources
Pain, 47, 82, 129, 139, 142-43
Pain killers, *see* Drugs, Over-the-counter (OTC)
Pap test, *see* Preventive tests
Pharmacist, *see* Health communication sources
Potency enhancers, *see* Drugs, Over-the-counter (OTC)
Prevention, 11-12, 53, 92, 104, 116-17, 148, 155, 208
Preventive tests
    Blood pressure, 64, 65, 80, 90, 114, 126
    Bone scan, 45, 64, 90, 99
    Cholesterol, 45, 64, 90, 114, 126
    Hemoglobin A1c, 64, 80, 90, 99, 126
    Mammogram, 45, 64, 114
    Pap test, 64, 90, 114, 126, 129
Product information, *see* Health communication sources

R

Relatives/friends, *see* Health communication sources

S

Segmentations, Strategic Directions Group, Inc.
> Health
>> Disillusioned, 140, 144-45, 178-79, 181-2, 185-88, 217
>> Faithful Patients, 135, 139-44, 176-77, 182, 186, 217
>> Optimists, 143-44, 183-85, 188-89, 216-19
>> Proactives, 25, 135, 138-42, 175-76, 187-88, 216-21
> Health Compliance
>> Cost-concerned Cynics, 170-72, 185, 186-87
>> Informed Avoiders, 163-66, 170, 180-185
>> Resentful Compliers, 163, 167-71, 178-79, 181, 187-89
>> Trusting Believers, 136, 161-66, 175, 178-79, 185
> Health Information
>> Confused Compliants, 148, 156-58, 176, 181, 185-86
>> External Health Actives, 136, 158-60, 176, 180, 182-83
>> Fearful Listeners, 152-54, 177-78, 181-83
>> Internal Health Actives, 154-56, 176-77, 180, 188
>> Self-directed Positives, 150-52, 184
>> Uninvolved Fatalists, 25, 146-50, 175-77, 181-82, 184

Sinus problems, *see* Diseases
Skin lotions for dry skin, *see* Drugs, Over-the-counter (OTC)
Skin ointments for irritations, *see* Drugs, Over-the-counter (OTC)
Skin ointments for pain, *see* Drugs, Over-the-counter (OTC)
Sleeping pills, *see* Drugs, Over-the-counter (OTC)
Sodium, *see* Food components
Spouse, *see* Health communication sources

Stroke, *see* Diseases
Sugar, *see* Food components

T

Targeting, 2-4, 17-18, 28, 50, 92, 104, 136, 199, 202, 208
Television shows, *see* Health communication sources

U

Uninsured, 44, 61, 100, 125, 127, 130
    see also Health insurance, No health insurance

V

Veterans Administration (VA), *see* Health insurance
Videos, see Health communication sources
Vitamins, *see* Drugs, Over-the-counter (OTC)

W

Wellness
    Coach/counselor, 4, 191, 195-196,200
    Employee wellness programs, 192-93, 195, 197-200,
        203, 209
    Plans, 25, 196
    Professional, 195

INDEX OF AUTHORS

Cross, R.M. 23
Cutler, David 205

D

Davenport-Firth, David, 202, 204
Davis, Karen, 10, 13
Davis, Robert, 203
Dewan, Shaila, 56
Dodge, Robert D., 29-31
Douglas, William, 56-7

E

Eastman, Peggy, 106
Erikson, Erik, 31

F

Farhat, Sally, 70
Flegal, Katherine, 50
Francis, David R., 12
Francis, Leo, 202
Fuhrmans, Vanessa, 83, 131-2

G

Gaman, Walter, 55
Geiger, Kim, 131
Geraghty, Estella M., 105
Gilmer, Todd P., 131
Ginsburg, Paul, 7
Goetzel, Ron Z., 204
Griffin, S. J., 72

H

Hendrick, Bill, 71
Herzlinger, Regina E., 7, 11-13
Hesse, Bradford W., 104
Himmelstein, David, 127
Hirth, Richard, 205
Holt, Cheryl L., 93

J

Jauhar, Sandeep, 82
Johnson, Avery, 132

K

Keehan, Sean P., 12-13, 209
Kellerman, Arthur L., 209
Kelly, R.B., 23
Kolbert, Elizabeth, 56-7
Kottke, Thomas, 53, 57
Kronick, Richard G., 131

L

Lee, Albert, 83
Lee, Vernon J., 71-2
Levinson, Wendy, 203-4
Levit, Katharine R., 12-13

M

Machlin, Steven R., 72
Mackey, Amy, 92
Marks, James S., 51